Improving Online Presentations

Can Cemal Cingi • Nuray Bayar Muluk
Cemal Cingi

Improving Online Presentations

A Guide for Healthcare Professionals

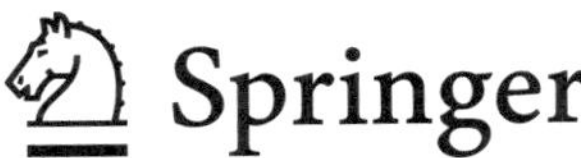

Can Cemal Cingi
Faculty of Communication Sciences
Anadolu University
Tepebaşı/Eskişehir, Türkiye

Nuray Bayar Muluk
Department of Otorhinolaryngology
Faculty of Medicine, Kirikkale University
Kirikkale, Türkiye

Cemal Cingi
Department of Otorhinolaryngology
Faculty of Medicine, Eskişehir Osmangazi
University
Eskisehir, Türkiye

ISBN 978-3-031-28330-7   ISBN 978-3-031-28328-4   (eBook)
https://doi.org/10.1007/978-3-031-28328-4

This Springer imprint is published by the registered company Springer Nature Switzerland AG
The registered company address is: Gewerbestrasse 11, 6330 Cham, Switzerland

Preface

Health sciences develop at a prodigious rate, creating a continuous demand for presentations of high quality and relevance. Presentations in healthcare and medicine are unique in the extent to which they influence daily healthcare practice. They are often the main way in which doctors and other healthcare professionals update their skills and knowledge. This book considers the needs of all presenters, from the beginning practitioner, facing an eager crowd with a heavy heart and shaking knees, to the experienced veteran, looking to polish his or her presentations skills in the new and challenging online arena.

This book is for anyone who has ever attended an unforgettable presentation, whether that indelible memory was created by an hour of torture and boredom or an hour of uplift, inspiration and enlightenment. We will teach you how to make your audience sit up and listen, relish your every word and go away feeling wiser and more satisfied.

But what is the secret of successful presenting? Is it pure chance, or is there a formula you can follow to ensure a good result every time? We strongly believe it is the latter. Knowing all the ingredients well and combining them skilfully is what makes a master chef and the same is true of a master presenter. We will show you everything, from audience analysis to handling the trickiest questions.

What makes this book so unique, though, is the great attention paid to achieving presenting excellence in an online environment. Online audiences are very different from face-to-face groups. Understanding why this is so gives presenters the insight they need to succeed virtually, as well as face-to-face. Medicine and healthcare are truly international enterprises and online presentations have a huge role to play in bringing together practitioners from all across the globe. Thus, every practitioner needs to be knowledgeable about virtual presentations.

Of course, in preparing this book, I have relied on the support and encouragement of many people, both professionally and personally. I owe an enormous debt of gratitude to Mrs Nuray Bayar Muluk, who has helped me and sustained me throughout my academic career to date, acting as a mentor, wise friend and even a sister or mother to me.

My father, Cemal Cingi, has also been a constant sustaining force behind the preparation of this book. Of course, no son likes to admit his father knows best, nor would ever admit that, but I will happily agree that his superior experience and persuasive explanations have enormously enriched both the content and form of this book. Nor can I omit mention of the many helpful insights, suggestions and ideas that came from other members of the Cingi Clan, either. My mother, Didem, and brother, Alp, both showed me many times what good communication really looks like in practice. They have a knack for resolving writer's block and keeping my spirits high in difficult times.

Ours is an unusual family. My father is a surgeon, my mother a dentist and I am an academic specializing in communication. This sometimes gives us very different perspectives, but this book has been a wonderful opportunity to combine these facets, by focusing on one vital part of healthcare communication—the presentation.

It only remains for me to wish you, the reader, a happy experience of online presenting. Be sure to keep this book by your side as you explore the world of virtual presenting. After all, nobody is born a perfect presenter. By acting on the advice here, though, any presenter can ensure they constantly improve their practice. And is not that what medicine is really all about, constant improvement?

Happy Presenting!

Tepebaşı/Eskişehir, Turkey   Can Cemal Cingi

Contents

What Leads to Success in Presenting? Consider the Audience, Subject and Time You Have Available

1.1 Introduction

Everybody has been unfortunate enough to attend a thoroughly tedious presentation at least once. Yet, if you have ever been at a presentation that has informed you, excited you or even inspired you, you will know that there is a world of difference between the presentation you have never forgotten (for all the wrong reasons) and the presentation you will never forget (for all the right reasons). So what creates that difference? There are a number of key elements to consider, as follows.

1.1.1 The Topic

Be Passionate About the Topic Unless you convey your own excitement and interest in a topic, your audience's reaction will never be more than lukewarm. If you feel bored yourself, how can you expect the listeners to be interested? Focus on what draws you to the topic, the aspect that got you involved. It is your duty as a presenter to bring passion and interest to the topic. Never settle for mumbling and bumbling your way through.

Know your topic inside out. Ensure you are well-informed on the topic and avoid making assumptions. Read up on the topic, note the key points and make up your mind on issues related to the topic.

Consider the Presenting Context You will need to tailor your content depending on who you will be presenting to. Suppose that you are talking about a newly released drug. The way you talk about it will differ depending on the audience involved. Journalists will have very different expectations from a group of pharmacology research scientists. The content needs to fit the context.

Think About Why This Topic Was Chosen You should be able to justify why the audience should give up their time to listen to you on this subject.

Ensure there is a single "take home message". After reflecting on any topic, there should emerge a central, organising idea that pulls the whole topic together and that you want your audience to grasp. By bringing a topic down to its bare essentials, you make it memorable for the audience [1].

1.1.2   The Format

Time limits exist for a good reason. Even if your brief does not include a time limit, a wise presenter knows to introduce one. At least 25% of the allocated time should be left to allow questions from the audience. In the worst-case scenario, where there are no questions, nobody ever blames a speaker for finishing a little early. The time limit is helpful in ensuring the presentation remains properly "on topic".

Plan what you want to say first. Never begin by starting to create your slides, whether you are using PowerPoint, Impress, Prezi or some other presenting software. That should only begin once you have a clear road map in mind for how you plan to discuss the elements of the topic. Ideas should first be sketched out and the connections between the elements noted. Some presenters like to create a mind map first, others create lists. More than one structure may well be possible. Experiment. This stage can be done equally well on paper, or with specialist software (Coggle, Mindly, Visio, etc.)

PowerPoint and Its Competitors (Impress, etc.) are the de facto industry standard, whatever individual presenters may feel about the issue. However, a standard need not restrict your presenting style. To avoid the infamous "death by PowerPoint" scenario, the marketing guru Guy Kawasaki advises the following format: **10** slides in **20** min with text in at least a **30**-point font.

Slides Should Help Rather Than Hinder the Flow of the Presentation Indeed, some presenting formats, such as Ignite or Pecha Kucha, are set up so that the next slide appears automatically after a definite time limit (15 s for Ignite). The intention is to force the speaker to keep going at a rapid pace.

Images Offer a Chance to Inspire Your Audience Do not waste this potential by over-reliance on stock images or readily available clip art. Presenters can use photographs they already own or license them from various sources. Flickr has many photographs licensed under a Creative Commons agreement. For other images, pay attention to licensing requirements, particularly for public presentations [1].

1.1.3   Contents of the Presentation

Presentations should be as **brief, pleasant and relevant** as possible. The presentation should follow this maxim overall. Choose words that are easily understood and not excessively technical. Remain concise and on-topic.

Use Storytelling Techniques Audiences respond well to a clear narrative. Narration is a genre that anybody can create and readily understand. Ask yourself what story lies behind the topic of your presentation.

Provide concrete examples to illustrate the key points. Audiences may struggle to understand a presentation that does not seem to relate well to their ordinary expectations and reality. Keep providing illustrative examples so that the ground seems more familiar to your listeners.

Think in advance about what your audience may ask you. The late writer Donald Murray advised that writing well involves anticipating the questions that form in a reader's mind as the story progresses and presenting the answers at that point. This philosophy is equally applicable to presenting. The objective is not to strangle discussion during the questions (far from it), but to ensure that your listeners are not left missing a key piece of information to understand the topic.

Decide what can be skipped if necessary. Presentations rarely go 100% according to plan, with disruptions due to latecomers or questions that call for detailed answers. Leave some room in your schedule to accommodate disruption by identifying what can safely be omitted, should time be short [1].

1.1.4   Preparing Yourself to Present

Familiarise yourself with the equipment and software. Make sure you know how to skip a slide, hide your notes, go back or forward and turn the projector on or off. If you embed files, make sure your application can access them. Presentation software, such as PowerPoint, has many keyboard shortcuts that can save you a lot of time when presenting.

Practice makes perfect. Doing a dry run (in front of the mirror) is essential to sounding professional and knowledgeable on your topic. Go over the presentation several times on the evening before and the morning of the presentation. However, avoid over-rehearsing, since this can make you appear stilted. The ideal situation is to know the subject well enough to be able to present without any aids at all. This situation may actually occur if there is a power cut, for example.

Consider what you will wear to present. At the risk of stating the obvious, it is clearly essential to have your speaking outfit ready in advance. Failure to have it completely ready can damage your concentration on the day of the presentation and may cause additional anxiety and loss of time. The outfit should be appropriate to the setting, whether formal or more casual.

Familiarise yourself with the venue for the presentation. Whenever it is feasible, presenters should become familiar with details of the venue. How large is it? Is it generally a comfortable environment? To what extent will you need to project your voice to be heard clearly? Even if the presenter cannot completely control some factors, knowing about them in advance allows precautions to be taken. Plan any interactive activities (such as questions or polls) after taking into consideration the physical environment. It is hard to hear a question from the back of a large lecture theatre if there is no portable microphone available.

Ensure your information is up-to-date. When gathering the information for a presentation, it is essential to check the source of facts, but some details are more liable to last minute alterations than others. Sales figures may be worse or better than the predictions, a new product may suddenly be launched, or a new manager may be appointed.

1.1.5   On the Day Itself

Ensure You Take Everything You May Need With You Do not place reliance on somebody else having remembered to leave a laptop set up for you. It is easy to forget to bring the cables to connect devices and even easier to forget a network password allowing access to a corporate or academic institution's intranet. Carry spare electronic copies of the presentation, as well as paper notes, for cases where the power fails.

Time Your Arrival Carefully You need to be focused, so this is the time to take a comfort break, drink some water (but not coffee or chocolate as they can provoke coughing) and warm up in good time for the presentation. Check the audiovisual equipment is in good working order.

Warm Up Before Presenting A wide variety of techniques are available that help with both the physical and psychological aspects of presenting. They are often used by actors to conquer the so-called stage fright and to prepare the voice so as to avoid vocal strain. There are some useful videos on the YouTube channel, hpbizanswers HP, which you may wish to watch.

Establish a connection (rapport) with the audience. A live presentation is a performance, not a mechanical repetition. Whilst presenting, be alert to feedback the audience is providing, especially through body language, such as shifting in the seats, sitting forward, smiling or frowning and so on. Try to sense the mood of the audience and adjust your delivery accordingly.

Share the message and keep the conversation going. Consider how you can share your slides with the audience following the actual presentation. There are a number of services that allow you to share slides, including SlideShare, Google Slides and PowerPoint Online. If you send a follow-up communication to the attendees, you can ask for any extra questions and solicit feedback on your ideas.

1.2   How to Plan for a Presentation

Being asked to present can feel very daunting. There seem to be a vast number of factors to consider. However, by approaching preparation of the presentation in a systematic way, you can ensure the job steadily proceeds to completion [2]. The following are the stages needed in preparing a presentation.

1.2.1   Initial Stage: Analysing the Potential Audience

The first task is to gather as much information about the potential audience as possible. This information lets you anticipate what kind of presentation will be needed and what sort of expectations there may be. Try to find out about the listeners' background, their areas of interest and any attitudes you might expect them to already hold.

1.2.2   Second Stage: Choosing a Topic

The next task is to identify a subject that both you and your potential listeners are likely to be engaged by. Not only does this mean that the audience are more likely to respond in a positive way to the presentation, it also means that the research phase will feel less onerous for you, as the presenter [2].

1.2.3   Third Stage: Setting the Aims for the Presentation

Having selected an appropriate subject for the presentation, you should try to define in one sentence what the aims of the presentation are. There should be a clear learning goal. The goal of the presentation is partly determined by how long you have to speak for and how knowledgeable your audience is already likely to be. Having a clearly defined aim is useful for maintaining focus in the research phase and whilst deciding on exactly what the content should be [2].

1.2.4 Assembling the Content You Intend to Present

1.2.4.1 Fourth Stage: Filling Out the Main Body of the Presentation

Once the aims have been clearly delineated, you can decide on the volume of information that the presentation will contain. The background knowledge about the likely attendees should guide you in knowing how detailed the content needs to be. The aim is to avoid the extremes of being either much too simplistic or way above the heads of your audience [2].

The essential concepts of the presentation are found in the body of the presentation. For each concept you introduce, if you can provide an illustration of how the concept applies, you will more easily convince your audience of the validity of what you are claiming. There are various ways to enhance the basic message of a presentation, such as [2]:

- Providing data and facts which confirm your interpretation.
- Quoting the opinions of experts in that field.
- Providing examples from your own experience.
- Describing situations in a way that makes them come alive to the audience.

Of course, these techniques should be used in a varied manner. Too much supportive evidence, rather than convincing an audience, may leave them feeling overwhelmed and confused. Likewise, a skilled presenter avoids making a presentation turn into a set of anecdotes that lead nowhere.

1.2.4.2 Fifth Stage: Decide How to Introduce the Topic and How You Will Conclude the Presentation

With the body of the presentation complete, the next step is to think how to introduce the presentation and how to bring it to a close. The introduction serves the key function of getting your audience engaged. The conclusion needs to remind the audience what they have heard and what the "take home message" is. In essence, you tell your listeners the same ideas three times—in the introduction, the body and the conclusion [2].

The introduction is a key time to engage the audience and provoke their curiosity. Failure to do so at the beginning means you will face an uphill struggle in the body of the presentation. The following are all ways to build audience engagement from the start: [2]

- Relate the topic to what your audience is already interested in, believes or wishes to achieve.
- You might pose a challenge at the beginning, to get the audience wondering about the topic.
- Tying the topic to lived experience makes it more relatable.
- Humour is a powerful tool.
- Cartoons attract attention, as do images that are full of colour.

- Use language that aims to inspire and challenge the audience.
- Show the audience something that they have never seen before.

The introduction should make clear exactly what subject you will address and why. This is important in directing the attention of the listeners and guiding them through the ideas of the main body.

Use your conclusion to reiterate the key concepts covered earlier. It is important to be realistic about the fact that an audience cannot be expected to retain the presentation in detail. The aim is for them to retain salient points. By reiterating the key messages, you make it more likely they take home the right message [2].

1.2.5   Practise Your Presentation Before You Deliver It

1.2.5.1   Sixth Step: Practice Makes Perfect

Although people often expend a large amount of effort in preparing the contents of a presentation, it is surprisingly common for people to overlook the need to practise the delivery. However, a practised delivery means fewer hesitations or repetitions and makes the speaker appear much more authoritative. Practising delivery is also essential to ensure you can adequately cover the material in the available time.

You should also ask yourself how you would prefer to deliver your presentation. You might choose to memorise the speech, make use of prompt cards or notes or even read from a pre-prepared script. It is also possible to use a combined approach. The following sections outline the pros and cons of each of these techniques [2].

1.2.6   Delivering a Speech from Memory

The key advantage to this method is that it keeps your hands free and means you do not need to handle notes or cards while speaking. Presenters who speak from memory can make use of the whole stage and can look at the audience rather than glancing down at notes. The technique does, however, suffer from several drawbacks. Delivering a memorised speech may sound somewhat unnatural and it is fairly easy to misremember a key point, omit an important section or suddenly have your memory go blank. Thus, if you do decide to memorise your speech, do not forget to keep some prompt cards ready to use in case your memory lets you down [2].

1.2.7   Using Prompt Cards or Notes

Speaking with the aid of prompt cards or notes is a popular choice. Usually presenters prefer to have a set of notes separate from the presentation itself, but it is also feasible to add speaker notes to your presentation in some applications, such as PowerPoint. Having some notes to support you can allow a more natural and spontaneous style of delivery and does not prevent the speaker from establishing intermittent eye contact with the audience. One potential disadvantage of speaking from notes rather than having memorised exactly what you want to say is that you may express yourself less well than you would have wished to [2].

1.2.8   Reading from a Script

To make use of this method, you need to prepare an exact script, which you can then read out to your audience exactly as it is written. This gives you the advantage of being able to consider the precise way you want to express an idea in advance, but it has the downside that such delivery can easily sound flat or mechanical. If you read from a script, you will need to make eye contact with your audience from time to time and ensure that you read in an expressive and lively way to engage the audience in what you are saying [2].

1.2.9   Combining Delivery Techniques

In many cases, the optimal way to deliver a presentation may include all three methods. It has been suggested by many professional speakers that the initial section of the presentation and the conclusion should be committed to memory to allow a smooth, error-free start and ensure you leave the best impression. For parts of a presentation where you are already very familiar with your content, such as an anecdote based on personal experience, you may be able to use prompt cards only, to guarantee you do not omit a vital point. If there is a section where you need to be very precise, such as quoting a regulation or quoting another expert, it may be appropriate to read that section. It may ease the flow of your presentation if you highlight the fact that you intend to read a section by saying something like, "I would like to read you exactly what the Act states" [2].

1.3   Subjects for a Presentation

Perhaps the ideal way to choose a topic on which to present is to find a subject that you already know well and is of particular interest to your intended audience [3].

1.3.1   Selecting a Suitable Subject

For presentations where the aim is to provide specific information to your audience it can be a real challenge to select the most appropriate area on which to concentrate. However, selecting the most appropriate topic can be guided by thinking carefully about the following points:

- The intended aim of the presentation. Once you identify your aim, you know what you wish your listeners to take away from the presentation. If you wish to convince your audience, it is essential that you are clear what you want to convince them of!
- The intended audience. Think carefully about who your listeners will be. What is their average age, what background do they come from and what are they interested in already? Consider what attitudes your audience will come with and think about any social or cultural factors that may affect the message you deliver.
- What are your own interests? Consider where your passions lie and the topics with which you are most familiar. Choosing a subject you already find of interest will make the research phase of preparation easier and more enjoyable and will give the presentation an air of conviction.
- Be credible. A topic which is believable and a presentation that is well-researched and backed up with key information enhances your personal credibility as a presenter.
- Be concise. It is important to consider that audience's attention spans are relatively short. Some researchers even make the controversial claim that attention spans are decreasing. Whatever the truth of such claims, it is best to give your presentation a "punchy" title. Long titles may seem less interesting and give the impression the topic itself is unclear.

1.3.2 Advice on How to Convert a Potentially Dreary Topic into a More Exciting Presentation

It is easy to feel dispirited if the topic about which you need to present lacks immediate interest for you. In some cases a topic may be so brimful of technical detail that it might appear a thankless task to engage your audience in hearing about it.

This reaction is understandable, but a skilled presenter will realise that presentations only become dull if the presenters are themselves dull or uninteresting. With some consideration, even unpromising topics can be made more appealing and engaging for an audience.

- Focus on what relevance a topic has both for you and the audience. Why is it worth talking about?
- Do not present in a lifeless manner. You have your own personality and that personality can be used to add interest and liveliness to the presentation.
- Ultimately, topics in themselves are neutral, but there are more or less engaging ways to address them.
- Make your audience feel that they are participating in a discussion about a topic rather than being lectured to.
- Make use of rhetorical questions, whereby you pose a question before answering it yourself [3].

1.3.3   Examples of Topics that Are Readily Made into Presentations

The following are examples (chosen randomly) of topic titles that lend themselves well to being presented. Think about what makes these topics sound appealing and how they may be used as models for other attractive-sounding presentations [3].

1.3.3.1   Attractive Topics for a Presentation
- *A Contemporary View on Heroes in Ancient Medicine*
- *How Antidepressants Affect the Human Brain*
- *Poor Nutrition and Attractiveness*
- *Can Music Improve Your Mental Health?*
- *From Traditional Herbal Remedy to Approved Treatment*
- *The Benefits of Sports for Health*
- *Productivity In Pandemics*

1.3.3.2   Subjects that Offer Good Potential for Presentations
- *Do the Media Promote Healthy Nutrition?*
- *Do Beauty Contests Boost or Harm Women's Self-esteem?*
- *Is religion helpful for improving health?*
- *How Gambling Affects Mental Health*
- *Authoritative Or Authoritarian? Which Doctors Achieve Most?*
- *How the Health System Can Get Better*
- *Anticipating and Avoiding Epidemic Diseases*
- *Beating Sleeplessness*
- *Healthy Interactions Between Children and their Pets*

1.3.3.3   Themes for a Mini-Presentation
- *Using Apps to Boost Your Fitness*
- *Advices for First-Time Fliers*
- *Simple, Tasty and Healthy Breakfast in 5 Min*
- *Beat the Procrastination Trap and Stay Healthy*
- *Danger! Social Media Can Ruin Your Nutrition*
- *The Best and Worst of Online Fitness Classes*
- *Go with Your Gut Feelings*

1.3.3.4   Enjoyable Topics to Present
- *Dance for Wellbeing*
- *Elite and Exclusive Healthy Food*
- *Diets that Teens Will Love*
- *Secrets People in Healthy Relationships Know*
- *What Can Art Therapy Do for You?*
- *The Differences between Trainer and Chiropractor*
- *Can Artificial Intelligence Improve Health?*
- *Tips and Tricks to Have the Best Body Shape*

1.3.3.5 Presenting about Health and Safety
- *Frequent Errors in Remaining Safe*
- *Addressing Stress at Work and Becoming More Ergonomic*
- *Essential Precautions to Avoid COVID*
- *Dealing with Violent Situations*
- *Electrical and Fire Safety*
- *Accidents at Work. What to Report, How to Stop Them and Who Is Liable?*
- *Safely Preventing Heat Exhaustion*
- *Frequently Seen Injuries at Work*
- *Communicating Safely and Effectively*
- *Responding Effectively in an Emergency*

1.3.3.6 Topics Which Are Easy to Present
- *Are GMOs Bad for Healthy Living?*
- *Improving the Effectiveness of Health Services to Older Adults*
- *Never Be Late Again*
- *How Does Globalization Affect People Worldwide?*
- *The Benefits of Smiling Therapy on Your Mental Health*
- *3D Printing in Medicine*
- *Language Learning Through the Power of Music*
- *Helping the Genius Child*

1.3.3.7 Presenting Controversial Subjects
There are inexhaustible subjects of controversy, especially on the Internet. Although these topics may easily generate interest, if you intend to present on the subject, be sure to be well-informed first to avoid making a negative impression on your audience [3].

Some Potentially Controversial Presentation Areas
- *Termination of Pregnancy—A Woman's Choice?*
- *Multicultural Societies and Their Benefits*
- *Is Electronic Voting Safe and Secure?*
- *Should the Public Own Guns?*
- *How Ethical Is Journalism?*
- *Do Patients Have the Right to Die?*
- *Should We Have Capital Punishment?*
- *Do Automatic Minimum Terms for Crimes Work?*
- *The Use of Torture During Interrogation*
- *IsIit Time to Get Rid of Electoral Colleges?*
- *Can Global Peace Really Exist?*
- *Homosexual Marriage*
- *Should Child Criminals Be Treated the Same as Adults?*
- *Outlawing Vivisection*
- *How Free Should Speech Be?*
- *Bans, Blockades and Divestment*

- *Is Insanity an Excuse for Crime?*
- *Tobacco Control*

Suitable Controversial Topics for Teenagers to Present
- *Casual Sex and Teenagers*
- *Blocking Pornographic Websites and Content*
- *Depression and Mental Health Problems in Adolescence*
- *Who Is Responsible for Teenage Suicides?*
- *Informing Teenagers About Drug Misuse*
- *Teenagers with Anorexia or Bulimia*
- *At What Age Should Teenagers be Allowed to Drink Alcohol?*
- *Should Parents Decide Who Their Teenage Children Date?*
- *The Pros and Cons of Virtual Medical Education*
- *What Fast Food Does to Teenagers*
- *How Does Being a Fan Affect Adolescent Development?*
- *Why Teenagers Need to Know About Health*
- *Do We Need School Uniforms and a Dress Code for Student Psychology?*
- *Providing Contraception to Underage Young People*

1.3.4   Suitable Topics for Presentations in Academic Institutions

As with any presentation, there is a need to identify topics which are both informative and enjoyable to learn. However, when presenting to children, remember that their ability to concentrate is usually less than adults. The following sections present ideas for topics that may be used in schools, colleges or higher education [3].

1.3.4.1   Presentations in Universities
- *Healthcare Provision and Regulation*
- *Should Everybody Be able to Connect to the Internet for Free?*
- *Do Video Games Affect our Mental Performance?*
- *Eradicating Poverty*
- *The Effects of Social Media*

1.3.4.2   Presentation Ideas for Use in Secondary Schools
- *Do TV Adverts Really Affect Us?*
- *Getting the Most Out of Volunteering*
- *Virtual Reality and What It Means for Us*
- *Does a Glass Ceiling Harm Business?*
- *Global Warming*

1.3.4.3   Suitable Brief Topics for School Students to Present
- *Using Social Media in School*
- *Learning to Respect and Work with Diversity*
- *What is Gentrification?*

- *Getting Accepted Into a Non-paid University*
- *Cinema Through the Ages*

1.3.5 Scientific Presentations

The most frequently requested presentations are usually those involving science. This applies to both students and teachers. The following are suggestions for topics that may be presented [3].

1.3.5.1 Suitable Topics for Physics Presentations
- *Is Physics Based on Experiments or Theory?*
- *Why Do We Need Physics?*
- *Newton's Third Law—The Key to Everything?*
- *Why We All Need the Formulae of Physics*
- *Who Leads the Way? Mathematicians, Physicists or Other Scientists?*
- *How Does Physics Prove Knowledge?*
- *Challenging Classroom Situations in Physics*
- *The Key Concepts of Physics* [3]

1.3.5.2 Suitable Topics for Chemistry Presentations
- *What Was the Philosopher's Stone in Alchemy?*
- *Nobel Prize-Winning Chemists*
- *The Terrifying Reality of Chemical Warfare*
- *Which Water Is the Best?*
- *Engaging Young Students in Chemistry*
- *The Biochemical Story of Hair*
- *Missing Nutrients and Their Effects on Human Health*
- *Handling Chemicals Safely* [3]

1.3.5.3 Suitable Topics for Biology Presentations
- *Interdisciplinary Studies Are the Future of Biology*
- *Avoiding GMO Food That May Damage Your Health*
- *How to Live to Be 100*
- *Dust Allergies*
- *Is Clean Drinking Water Essential for Life?*
- *Eating Well, Exercising Often and Living Healthily*
- *Do Vaccines Change Our Genes?*
- *Which Indoor Plants Most Improve Air Quality?*

1.3.5.4 Suitable Topics for Geology Presentations
- *Seismic Events as Dynamic Drivers of Geology*
- *Geomorphology: Where Geology and Geography Meet*
- *Astrogeology—The Geology of the Cosmos*
- *The Geological Progression: Bedrock to Holocene*

- *Dating Geological Events Relatively and Absolutely*
- *Geological Techniques and Theories*
- *Geodynamics: How the Core and the Crust Interact*
- *Geological Microstructure: How Rocks Are Deformed at the Microscopic Level*

1.3.5.5 Suitable Topics for Astronomy Presentations

- *How do Astronomy and Astrology Differ?*
- *Could There Be Life on Mars?*
- *How the Milky Way Formed and How We Know*
- *Is Astronomy Only About Stars?*
- *Astronomy as a Stand-alone School Subject*
- *Why Don't More Students Choose Astronomy?*
- *When the Sun Stops*
- *Astronomy Is Vital for the Future of Humanity*

1.3.5.6 Suitable Topics for Technology Presentations

- *Better Quality of Life Through Technology*
- *Technological Progress in Treating Cancer*
- *Technologically Smart Criminals*
- *Artificial Intelligence: Advantages and Risks*
- *Managing Your Time Online*
- *The Progress of Technology—Mediaeval to Contemporary*
- *How Quickly Does Technology Catch on in Developing Countries?*
- *Getting Away from the Internet*

1.3.5.7 Suitable Topics for Multimedia Studies Presentations

- *How to Classify Different Multimedia on their Features*
- *Getting Creative with Multimedia*
- *What Are Online Multimedia Like?*
- *Commercial Advantages of Multimedia*
- *Multimedia within Video Games*
- *Setting up Educational Programmes with Multimedia Features*
- *How to Specialise in Multimedia*
- *Multimedia in Science*

1.3.5.8 Suitable Topics for Culture Studies and Social Science Presentations

The following are some suggestions for topics of presentations in the field of social science [3].

Cultural Topics
- *Indigenous Cultures and Their Traditions*
- *What History Teaches Us About Culture and* Vice Versa
- *Cultural Intelligence Makes You More Successful*
- *Understanding Emigrant Cultures*

- *Why Cultural Knowledge Is Vital for Students*
- *Why Understanding Cultures Matters*
- *Is Being Cosmopolitan Always a Good Thing?*

Sociology
- *The Ideal Books for Beginning Sociology Students*
- *What Makes Sociological Research Different?*
- *Empirical Studies in Sociology*
- *Social Effects and Their Causes*
- *Mathematical Sociological Techniques*
- *How to Analyse Societal Trends and Identify Patterns*
- *The Acquisition of Sociological Data* [3]

Leadership
- *How to Be the School President*
- *Leadership Skills a School President Requires*
- *Bringing Up Children Who Can Lead*
- *Are Leaders Born or Made?*
- *Leadership Duties*
- *How Families Sculpt Future Leaders*
- *How to Win a Leadership Scholarship* [3]

Moral Philosophy
- *Individual and Social Perspectives in Moral Philosophy*
- *Ethics in Domestic and International Politics*
- *Communicating Ethically on Social Media*
- *Acting Ethically in Business Relationships*
- *The Value of Understanding Etiquette*
- *The Ethics of Notorious Works of Art*
- *Knowledge of Business Ethics*

1.3.6   Suitable Topics for Healthcare Presentations

Many presentation subjects in the area of general or mental health are suitable to present in schools or elsewhere, but presenters must choose enjoyable topics and avoid making them over-complicated. The following are suggestions for topics to present that may be appropriate for such environments [3].

1.3.6.1   Suitable Topics for Psychology Presentations
- *Why Kindergartens Benefit from Psychological Input*
- *Colleges with the Best Reputation for Psychology*
- *Selecting the Most Appropriate Psychologist*
- *Exclusion and Its Effects on Children*
- *How Mental State Affects Your Productivity*

- *When to Seek Psychological Help*
- *Former Patients as Psychologists. Is It Possible?* [3]

1.3.6.2   Suitable Topics for Mental Health Presentations

- *Mental Fatigue as a Reason to Fail*
- *Social Media and How It Affects Your Mental Health*
- *Avoiding Depression and Recognizing the Warning Signs*
- *What Causes Mental Ill-Health?*
- *Interactions between Physical and Mental Health*
- *What To Do in a Nervous Breakdown*
- *The Benefits of Music for Mental Health* [3]

1.3.6.3   Suitable Topics for Presentations About Health

- *Why Do We Need Over-the-Counter Drugs?*
- *What Happens in an Allergic Reaction?*
- *Sports Which Make Your Healthier in Weeks*
- *Signs That Your Immune System Is Weak*
- *Should Cannabis Be Decriminalized?*
- *What Centenarians Know About Living Healthily*
- *Keeping Healthy in the Lead-Up to Exams*

1.3.6.4   Suitable Topics for Presentations About Nutrition

Why You Should Check What Products Contain
How Does Diet Affect Your Skin?
Working Out Nutritional Balance: Protein, Carbs and Fat
Eating Well on a Restricted Diet
The Dangers in Sports Diets
Advantages of Becoming a Nutritionist
Nutrition and Its Effects on Success

1.3.6.5   Suitable Topics for Nursing Presentations

- *A Career in a Growing Field: Nursing*
- *Safe and Wise Use of Analgesics*
- *Keeping Patients Safe During Nursing Interventions*
- *What Should a Health Check-Up Include?*
- *Nursing the Mentally Ill*
- *Post-surgical Recovery Nursing*
- *Learning from Clinical Placements*

1.3.6.6   Suitable Topics for Dentistry Presentations

- *Looking after Infant Teeth*
- *How Molar Teeth Are Extracted*
- *Are the Third Molars Essential?*
- *What Does Chewing Gum Do To Dental Enamel?*

- *What Causes Mouth Cancer and How Is It Treated?*
- *Suitable Diets for Patients with Retainers*

1.3.6.7   Suitable Topics for Medicine Presentations
- *How to Summon Emergency Help*
- *Substance Misuse Medicine*
- *Medications That Are More Addictive Than Commonly Realized*
- *First Aid for Stab Injuries*
- *Reasons to Operate on Patients*
- *Traditional, Alternative and Allopathic Drugs*
- *Avoidance of Sporting Injury*
- *Non-drug Treatment of Insomnia*
- *Anti-Ageing Pills—Know the Dangers*
- *Should You Donate Your Organs After You Die*
- *Are Euthanasia and Suicide Linked?*
- *Stopping Children Becoming Obese*
- *Advantages and Disadvantages of Genetic Engineering*
- *Multiple Methods for Healthcare Improvement*
- *Why Plastic Surgery Requires Clear Regulations*

1.3.7   What Types of Topics Are Suitable in a Business or Management Context?

The choice of a business or management topic to present is guided by the need to appear confidently knowledgeable about the topic when you present. The following are some suggestions for suitable presentations [3].

- *Topics Related to Strategy*
- *SWOT Analysis*
- *Why Ethical Companies Have Higher Sales*
- *Doing Business Across Borders*
- *Customers Expect Empathy*
- *Most Recent Market Openings*
- *Where Do We Go From Here?*
- *Development and Success in Online Business*

1.3.7.1   Business Topics that May Be More Challenging
- *Sharing Contentious Information*
- *Managing Sexual Harassment Claims in the Workplace*
- *Dealing with Micro-aggression*
- *Managing Crowds and Ensuring Safety*
- *Dealing with Conflicts Amongst Employees*
- *Communicating Across Different Cultures*

- *Dealing Constructively with Criticism*
- *Dealing with Workplace Disagreements*
- *Reacting to Hostility*

1.3.7.2   Topics for Managers

- *How to Manage the New Hire*
- *Successful Supervision*
- *Developing Your Management Skills*
- *Developing Staff Who Report to You*
- *Mentoring Other Employees*
- *Feedback Matters*
- *Essential Insights for New Managers*
- *Styles of Management*
- *Helping Newly Appointed Management Colleagues*
- *Becoming the Manager of Newly Created Divisions*

1.3.7.3   Topics to Inspire Your Audience

- *Remember Our Company's Past Successes*
- *What Do Our Customers Like About Us?*
- *How to Make Your Work Count*
- *Meaningful Careers*
- *Being an Employee with Passion to Succeed*
- *The Story of Our Company*
- *Experiences that Have a Positive Personal Impact*
- *Achieving for Your Community*
- *Inspiring Other People*
- *Remaining a Positive Employee*
- *Achieving All You Can At Work*
- *Achieving Your True Potential*
- *Achieving What You Want*
- *Acquiring Positive Habits*

1.3.7.4   Topics for Continuous Training Courses

- *Preparing food safely*
- *Fundamental Topics in …*
- *Achieving Compliance in …*
- *Preventing Legal Liabilities*

1.3.7.5   Topics for Budding Entrepreneurs

- *Spotting Business Niches*
- *Why Every Company Needs Legal Advice*
- *Setting Up Small Companies*
- *Coming Up with Ideas for Novel Products*
- *Marketing Your Startup*
- *Entrepreneurial Thinking*

- *What To Do (and Not Do) When You Take on Your First Staff*
- *Getting Financial Backing for Your Startup*
- *The Pros and Cons of Virtual Businesses*
- *Crafting a Perfect Elevator Pitch*
- *The Culture of New Businesses*
- *Challenging the Existing Market*

1.3.7.6 Topics Concerning Productivity

- *Time Management Through Effective Deadlines*
- *Tools to Help You Manage Your Time Optimally*
- *Demonstrative Speaking and How It Helps Businesses*
- *Mental Hacks to Drive Greater Productivity*
- *What To Do (and Not Do) To Make Breaks Work for You*
- *Keeping Effective Working Habits*
- *Avoiding Afternoon Productivity Dips*
- *Achieving More in Less Time*
- *The Importance of Rest to Maximising Productivity*
- *Healthy Eating and Higher Productivity*
- *Overcoming the Barriers to Being Productive*

1.3.7.7 Topics Concerning Safety at Work

- *Stopping Fires Before They Start*
- *Emergency Management*
- *Preventing Workplace Illness*
- *Safe Operation of Machinery*
- *Avoiding Injuries at Work*
- *Dealing with Hazards in Workplace Environments*
- *Handling Chemicals Used in Manufacturing Safely*
- *Keeping Office Staff Safe*
- *Safety at Work for Non-employees*
- *Encouraging Workers to Adopt Healthy Habits*
- *The Creation of a Safe Environment at Work*
- *Preventing Trips, Slips and Falls*
- *Establishing a Safety-positive Culture at Work* [3]

1.4   Length of Presentations

There are a number of different factors which should be borne in mind when deciding on the optimal length of time a presentation should last. These factors include:

- The time slot allocated
- Who the audience will be and how familiar they are with the topic
- How complicated the topic to be discussed is
- What level of information needs to be given to the audience

The optimal length for a presentation has been the subject of several studies and experts generally agree that a presentation which lasts no longer than 8 min is ideal. This length offers the best return when the time invested in preparing the presentation is compared with the level of audience engagement with the presentation. Thus, in strictly rational terms, longer presentations suffer from decreasing marginal utility. This conclusion is, however, based on experience of delivering presentations to middle or executive level managers in corporate environments during the ordinary working day. It is essential when delivering and preparing a presentation to empathise with your audience. If, for example, you are presenting about a new product or service, you should think about what questions the audience are likely to have formed, and base the content on that, rather than simply running through the technical specifications of the product or service. A presentation of this kind needs to be customer- or market-focused. It may be a challenge to remove technical detail from a presentation to conform to what your audience wishes to hear, but this essential step should not be overlooked. Wherever possible, condense lengthy explanations into a single bullet point. Thus, rather than focusing on the optimal time duration for a presentation, it is better to pay attention to making the content as concise and relevant as possible. Every presentation should be tailored to fit the audience, guided by their interests and tastes [4]. A presentation fitting these criteria should not, by its very nature, be too long.

1.5   Presentation Skills in the Virtual Environment

There are a number of skills and techniques that are highly effective when delivering a presentation face-to-face, but which are no longer of value when presenting in an online environment. Yet there are also many techniques and skills which are as important and relevant in an online presentation as in a face-to-face setting. However, it is undeniable that the rise in teleconferencing, facilitated by the availability of applications, such as Zoom or Microsoft Teams, has altered the presenting landscape, potentially irreversibly. Thus, would-be presenters definitely now require knowledge of online presenting techniques. The following paragraphs discuss ways that online presenting differs from traditional formats and provides some suggestions for how to adapt to the new virtual world [5].

Many presenters question how it is possible to adapt the use of eye contact and gesture within the limitations of, say, a Zoom presentation. Whilst these are perfectly valid concerns, it is worth pointing out that, just as with more traditional formats, the key issue is which audience you will face, since this dictates the content. A well-constructed presentation is more important than the exact style of presentation. To ensure that you communicate the presentation well, you should begin by outlining a road map of the areas you intend to cover. This map involves a more structured approach than simply listing the topics and subtopics. A list on its own fails to attract the audience's attention [5].

After paying attention to how to structure the presentation, the next consideration is the style of presenting. In face-to-face presentations, one effective tactic is to establish eye contact with one member of the audience until you reach the end of your sentence, then switch eye contact to another person. This tactic is, unfortunately, not suitable for online presentations, so you may need to place more reliance on interaction. If you can see the participants and their names (as is usually the case on Zoom, for instance), and the audience is no more than 30 or 40 people, you can note the body language of a particular person and say, for example, "I guess your nodding your head indicates you agree, John", or something similar. In this way you should be able to interact with a half dozen or so members of the audience.

Online presenting also limits the extent to which you can gesture or use arm signals. The typical setup means you may need to remain in one place, since the webcam or camera is fixed. The field of view may be too narrow to show your gestures properly. There are some experimental virtual platforms that do capture gestures and permit more movement, but these are not commonplace so far. An alternative to add visual interest and variety in the presentation is to use some sort of "prop", such as a print-out, which you can then show in electronic form by sharing your screen. In this way, the audience can perceive your movement without becoming distracted by not being able to see the whole gesture [5].

Teleconferencing applications are designed to allow the audience to interact with the presenter. In this way they differ from broadcasting. You can encourage this type of interaction through polls, getting the audience to give a virtual thumbs up or thumbs down, or using the chat function. The interaction helps to offer a natural break in the presentation and to get the audience active. Ensure that these kinds of interactivity are also carefully planned to emphasise a particular learning point [5].

Furthermore, teleconferencing software also lets you share a video or audio clip. This can be used to bring in other opinions or to set the topic in a wider context. For example, in a presentation on healthcare, you might show a clip of another healthcare professional being interviewed on the same subject. This adds relevance to your presentation, showing the issue is widely discussed.

It is important to consider the time needed to play a clip. A 3-min clip will add 3 min to a presentation, so it should only be used if you can afford to use the time on the clip. Furthermore, presenters should ensure they know how to share the video. Few things are as distracting as a presenter who helplessly clicks everywhere on the screen with rising panic when the clip fails to be displayed.

Another key consideration when presenting virtually is the facial expression to adopt. Active listening (for example, when listening to a question) can be indicated by slightly raising the cheekbones, but without a full smile. This encourages the audience that they are being listened to as well as listening themselves. The resting face should convey enthusiasm and happiness to be present. If your face naturally falls into a glum look, you may find it helpful to practice in front of a mirror. If you are a member of the audience rather than the presenter, taking notes does allow you to keep looking down without appearing disconnected from the presentation [5].

References

1. Dodd C. How to make a successful presentation: 5 easy steps to perfection. https://www.articulatemarketing.com/blog/how-to-make-a-successful-presentation. Accessed 3 Oct 2021.
2. Steps in preparing a presentation. http://tutorials.istudy.psu.edu/oralpresentations/oralpresentations3.html. Accessed 3 Oct 2021.
3. Abhishek KG. 350+ presentation topics that will appeal to any audience. 2020. https://www.orai.com/blog/presentation-topics/. Accessed 3 Oct 2021.
4. Ideal presentation duration. https://bharatgrouponline.com/about-us/knowledge-center.htm. Accessed 3 Oct 2021.
5. Spaeth M. Presentations and presentation skills in the age of virtual meetings. 2020. https://www.forbes.com/sites/forbesagencycouncil/2020/11/25/presentations-and-presentation-skills-in-the-age-of-virtual-meetings/?sh=201d000858fe. Accessed 3 Oct 2021.

2.1   Introduction

Face-to-face (hereafter referred to as F2F) is amongst the most effective of all ways to present and provide information to an audience at all fields from sales of basic home utensils to plastic surgery marketing. The reason for the high degree of communicative efficacy of this mode of presentation is that it involves simultaneous transmission of multiple cues to the intended meaning, unlike many other modes of communication. The principal mass media used in broadcasting, such as television, have the advantage that they can replicate many of the features of F2F, so that the audience can attend to non-verbal signals or cues, such as posture, body language, tone of voice and the expression on the presenter's face. A further advantage of F2F is the ease with which visual aids can be incorporated into a presentation and the way it facilitates use of rhetorical techniques (emphasis, pathos, mnemonics, etc.). These factors all come together to mean F2F presentations are often more memorable and convincing than other types.

In recent years, aesthetic surgery advertising and marketing activities have rapidly increased. Individuals go to different countries and have surgical procedures done because they are more accessible and more economical. This marketing strategy has developed the tendency to make the first meetings online but the final meetings face-to-face.

There have been studies examining the neurobiological basis for the effectiveness of F2F communicative events. These studies indicate that F2F induces greater synchronicity of the brain in participants than occurs in other types of communication scenario, which may help to explain why F2F encounters enable greater communicative efficacy and deeper exchange of meaning [1].

F2F presentations may occur in a variety of settings, ranging from presentations to an individual or small group through to a large public lecture. The venue for the presentation and the number of attendees will, of course, vary depending on the purpose for which the presentation was arranged.

There have been profound alterations in everyday communication which have come about through digitalization. These changes affect personal as well as business-related communication or aesthetic surgery marketing. It might be tempting to assume that the plethora or technologies which support virtual communication, such as e-mail, WhatsApp or Zoom, have put F2F communication in second place. However, the real situation is just the opposite—F2F is even more relevant now than ever before [2].

The preference for F2F is even marked amongst new entrants into the employment market, who grew up in a world of extreme digital connectivity and might be expected to be most used to virtual communication. Even amongst early career professionals, 68% express a preference for F2F communication in health care communication [2].

So, what are the reasons for still needing F2F in an era of plentiful digital communication technologies? And does F2F communication really have such an advantage over remote communication when speaking to business clients or a patient?

The next section will help to answer these questions. We introduce the reader to seven steps concerning best practice in F2F presentations/communication. These seven steps should make it easier to negotiate with success in business and establish an enduring relationship with someone [2].

2.2 The Seven Steps Involved in F2F Presentations

2.2.1 First Step: Know How F2F Communication Works Best

In this step, you should ask yourself what F2F really means as a concept. One pragmatic definition of F2F communication is that the participants in the communicative exchange can actually see each other. Despite being a useful first approximation to a definition of what F2F means, there are a number of complications to consider, as we will now see.

Another important point about F2F communication is that it refers to communication which does not rely on any particular technology to occur. The lack of an intervening or mediating technology means that the participants in the communicative exchange can more easily establish rapport and respect and lay the basis for a more enduring relationship.

Yet, as a business expands and covers an ever-larger geographical area, even crossing borders, F2F becomes increasingly less feasible, with other, less direct modes of communication, such as telephoning, e-mailing or use of text messaging replacing F2F communication and conferences being held virtually.

Despite the trend towards virtual communication, there is still a notable preference for F2F meeting, as this brings several advantages to the participants. Virtual communication suffers from the disadvantage of seeming impersonal to many people. Conversely, F2F meetings and presentations are more personal and may appear more authentic, which is helpful in creating a favourable impression of integrity. At present, no technology is able to fully replicate these positive effects [2].

The question then naturally occurs, why is F2F communication so markedly different to virtual communication? In what respects do F2F meetings differ from those conducted online?

The use of online meetings is generally reserved for situations where the attendees are geographically far apart or travel is difficult or expensive. Attendees may be in different time zones. The optimal situation in which to use teleconferencing is where you have already met the other attendees (whether clients, patients or colleagues) and have already established some kind of rapport.

Because of their limitations, online meetings should not be considered a default option or the main way of conducting meetings. Not only do they tend to be impersonal, but it has been shown that they are less time-efficient than F2F meetings, even threefold less so [3].

Online meetings also tend to prevent the attendees from properly seeing each other. This ability to see who you are talking to is an essential part in establishing a firm sense of rapport, on which an enduring patient–doctor relationship can be built.

It has also been reported by some businesses such as preoperative planning that a move away from F2F meeting resulted in a 17% fall in decision and related profit [4]. Some business leaders even go so far as to suggest that, rather than selecting which meetings should have the F2F format, all meetings should be F2F, unless the risk of not doing so is acceptably low [5].

Nonetheless, the COVID-19 pandemic demonstrated that there are occasions (such as lockdown or travel restrictions) when there is no alternative to virtual meetings. Online meetings, even though they are not a straight substitute for F2F meetings, may be still beneficial to build relationships with suitable clients, provided they are used in a way that takes account of their differences from F2F meetings [6]. There are now a number of publications which offer specific advice on business-to-business promotion strategies to use when working online [2].

2.2.2   Second Step: Find Out Who Is Making the Decisions

In the first step, the many advantages that come from F2F meetings were outlined, as well as why F2F is more effective for marketing than virtual meeting. However, this leaves a key issue unresolved, namely how to identify clients with whom it is worthwhile holding an F2F meeting. It is important to be clear how you will offer benefit to clients when you do meet them in-person.

One advantage that medical secretaries have currently is that there are a multitude of different platforms available where potential leads can be followed up. However, rather than meeting all your leads F2F, medical secretaries need to identify those surgery candidates with a realistic prospect for you. This step is known as **prospecting**.

It may be helpful when prospecting for suitable clients to establish a memorable figure or persona that can signify the target audience for the elective surgery marketing. Once the surgeons feel they understand fully what type of patient they are looking for, they can identify cases which may profit from their service or application they are promoting and work out which individuals in those occasions have the decision-making capacity. Prospecting involves noting who the stakeholders, key opinion leaders and gatekeepers are in the firm you wish to sell to, as well as obtaining details of how to contact those individuals.

Prospecting is a vital step in surgical recommendation and needs to be conducted in a planned fashion. The following are the steps required to accomplish the task in as efficient a manner as possible [2]:

Plastic surgery procedures with online interviews are getting more and more popular. Steps to undertake in prospecting:

1. Adopt a consistent strategy
   Ensure that you timetable a suitable slot every day in which you can work on prospecting. By consistently working on the task, medical secretaries can ensure they generate new leads and achieve a satisfactory promotion conversion rate.
2. Keep the objective in focus
   Begin by defining a set of objectives for the prospecting and divide the task up in such a way that every day you can advance towards your objective. Avoid getting sidetracked by other tasks and make sure your focus remains fixed on the daily objective you have set.
3. Employ a variety of methods
   Outline the prospecting techniques you aim to make use of an estimate how long each technique involves and the likely number of prospects you can reach with that particular method. Although it is sensible to use the technique most which offers the best return on time invested, you may need to switch techniques to ensure you reach all the possible prospects to reach more patients.
4. Prepare a promotion script
   You should have a script or template to follow when prospecting, so as to maximise the value of any communication with potential patients who are seeking for plastic procedures. It is a good idea to have thought about replies to likely objections. Keep developing the script in the light of the response shown by potential clients and ensure what you say has relevance to the person you are speaking to.
5. Keep your objective clearly in mind
   When prospecting, the objective is not to directly offer a certain procedure, then and there or to get into the details of a client's precise requirements. Prospecting is designed to give you an opening where you can promote an intervention that meets the patients need. Prospecting may be just in the first stage in cosmetic surgery marketing conversions.
6. Make cold calls as well as warm calls
   Even though cold calls often seem to produce disappointing results, the technique is a time-efficient way to begin a potential relationship in aesthetic field. Therefore, do not discount it from the techniques you plan to make use of.

   A warm call refers to one where there has been some prior contact between the aesthetic agent and the potential prospect. This contact may have been made through a referral from another client or perhaps via social media. There are several different types of warm call, which are discussed elsewhere [7].

7. Foster good relationships

   However well your plan for client prospecting is designed, it is inevitable that you will sometimes receive a negative response when you reach out to a prospect. Pay attention to how existing relationships can be nurtured and how you can most effectively add value to the relationships you are fostering

   It is vital not to lose sight of the main objective in prospecting. Prospecting is not intended to sell the services you represent, but rather to start new relationships, which may eventually lead to surgery.

   There are a number of excellent resources available which teach the best methods to hunt for new prospects. One such resource is Mark Hunter's book, "High Profit Prospecting" [8].

2.2.3   Third Step: Getting Meetings Booked in with Prospects

Following the initial hunt for likely prospects, the next stage is to book in an appointment with those people to allow you to present F2F.

The initial prospecting stages will have already involved obtaining background information on your prospects and what their likely requirements are. At this point, you should tailor the approach to this information and get in contact to book in a suitable F2F meeting to explain what you can do for that particular individual.

As mentioned earlier, both cold and warm calling offer a somewhat effective and easily undertaken method to identify potential prospects. However, these are not the only possible techniques which can be employed to obtain the crucial F2F meetings that you are aiming to set up. The following are some ways to establish contact with chief executive, C-level managers or other individuals with the authorization to agree to sales or surgery [2].

2.2.3.1   Five Particularly Effective Ways to Contact Prospects

1. Referral by Another Patient or Prospect

   It has been shown that the likelihood of a business-to-business (B2B) purchaser engaging with a doctor is increased five-fold when the introduction is made via a referral [9]. There is also a marked preference (73% of B2B decision-makers) for communicating with medical staff when introduced as a referral [10].

   It is surprising therefore to learn how rare it is for doctors to actively seek to be referred to other prospects. Research indicates that a request to be referred only occurred in 11% of cases [10]. Plastic surgeons would be wise to realise just how powerful referral is and to actively seek referrals from your network or other patients.

2. Cold-Calling

   Although many health care providers see cold-calling as an obsolete method, it has been shown that failure to use cold-calling actually shrank growth by as much as 42% [11].

   For a cold call to have a reasonable chance of success, the key is to adopt a positive attitude towards the technique. It is worth considering that no call to a prospect is truly "frozen", since you will already have conducted some initial research into the person to back up the reason for calling.

Another way of looking at cold-calling is from an added value perspective. View each contact as an opportunity to add value to a potential future business relationship through increasing the trust level. Each time you call, demonstrate your willingness to make the prospect's life easier.

3. Use of Social Media

Social media are extensively used by plastic surgeons as a way of establishing initial contact with prospects and making any subsequent communications less cold. Social media are highly beneficial in terms of letting prospects know about you and the surgeon you represent, in advance of getting into closer contact.

It was reported in an IDC white paper that there is extensive reliance on social media by individuals making decisions on purchasing for firms, including by C-level executives [12]. Furthermore, medical secretaries who employ social media techniques have a greater likelihood of keeping a continuous stream of prospects coming their way.

You should ensure that you connect with a prospect prior to attempts to reach that person via other techniques. This considerably warms up any subsequent interaction with that individual.

4. E-mailing

E-mailing is a technique that offers the advantages of not creating high pressure and being capable of high effectiveness. Nonetheless, e-mailing is a relatively complex technique and it is important that the specific way you use this channel corresponds appropriately to the prospect you are targeting.

There are a number of issues to consider when composing an e-mail to a prospective client, such as the existing level of familiarity between you. Writing to someone you have already connected with is different from writing to a complete stranger. Consider your objective—do you want to introduce the company as a whole or a specific product or service? What value will the e-mail offer the recipient? By considering these factors carefully and composing a well-thought-out e-mail, medical secretaries will greatly boost their chances of obtaining an F2F interview meeting.

What you write in the subject line of an e-mail is another critical issue. It has been estimated that an average office-based worker is sent more than 120 e-mails each day [13]. If you do not want your mail to remain amongst the growing pile of e-mails that remain unread, you will need to ensure it is personal to the prospective client and matches their interests.

Managing actually to speak to the key decision-maker in an organisation can be quite a complicated task; however, there are a number of useful resources available, offering advice on getting past gatekeepers, deciding on the best times to call and effectively combining e-mail with voicemail messages [2, 14].

2.2.4   Fourth Step: Getting Ready to Meet C-Level Executives

Having got this far, medical secretaries may feel some sense of relief, but it is still vital to ensure you brief yourself adequately for any F2F meetings with the surgeon you have been able to arrange, so as to achieve the optimal impact. There are a number of steps that should be taken to make sure that the meeting has the maximum chance to go according to the patient's wishes [2].

2.2.4.1   Steps to Take Prior to Attending F2F Meetings

1. Make Sure You Have Enough Background Information on the Prospective Surgical Client

   At an earlier stage, you will have already gathered some background information about the prospective client, but at this stage an additional search should be undertaken, to make sure you have not overlooked important details that may influence the client's reactions.

   It is a good idea to prepare in advance some questions you may use to elicit the problems the client is currently facing (the so-called pain points) and to appreciate what outcome they are hoping for. Similarly, think about what you may be asked and plan suitable responses, as well as having some case studies at your fingertips to illustrate how the procedure or surgery matches the client's expectations. It is vital that this preparation stage is not omitted; otherwise, the meeting will be neither client-focused nor informative to either party.

2. Define What You Hope to Achieve

   Identify what you feel should be the principal objective from the meeting. Naturally, for most medical presentations, the desired goal will be signing off on a surgery appointment.

   Nonetheless, it is worth remembering that the objective the salesperson has in mind may not exactly match that of the potential buyer. Thus, generally the principal goal should consist of becoming more familiar with the prospective client's pain points. This goal can be broken down into sub-goals.

   With a definite objective in mind and a reason for calling an F2F meeting, there is the maximum chance of the meeting progressing to a successful conclusion. Having a clear purpose means you will be able to direct the meeting along the lines you wish it to go. The lines to follow are dictated by the agenda, which is the next step to take to get ready.

3. Have an Agenda for Your Meeting

   In order to ensure the meeting makes the best use of the time available, you will need a clear agenda. The purpose of the meeting, any goals and objectives should already be clear from the previous steps. These can be added to the agenda.

   Write down how you intend to achieve the meeting's objectives, and this description will then be available as a plan for how to conduct the actual meeting. The following points are likely to appear in your notes:

- Ensure you know what the patient expects from the solution you are offering. How do they think it will add value?
- What return the patient anticipates getting if he/she decides to invest in what you have to offer.
- Would it be appropriate to set up a future meeting at which you can demonstrate the product or service in action such as previous results of previous surgery?
- As the meeting is happening, having this kind of list to hand will allow you to evaluate how you are performing. Are you covering the key points?
- Even though the agenda is a valuable guide, you will still need to be attentive to what the prospective client's requirements are and be flexible enough to deviate from the agenda if necessary. Avoid overstaying your welcome, however, as this wastes both your time and the prospective client's time.
- Wherever it is feasible, share the agenda you have prepared with your prospective client. In that way, they are aware of what the meeting will involve. An agenda gives the impression of efficiency and that you respect your prospect's valuable time.

4. Prepare a Contingency Plan

Despite your best efforts to plan precisely how the meeting will go, there is always a risk of the meeting not proceeding as you expected. This is the rationale behind preparing a backup plan in advance.

An example of the contingencies to consider is a late start or the meeting being curtailed, which may force you to leave out some topics or delay presenting them to another occasion. Furthermore, it is wise to prioritise the content that you most wish to discuss with your prospective client, if the meeting goes astray due to a long digression or lengthy debate about one specific point.

Alongside a backup plan, it is important to carry a hard copy (such as a paper copy) of any content you wish to present, in case of technological failure. Make sure any electronic devices are fully charged before presenting and carry physical copies of products if suitable. Before setting off for a meeting, ensure the prospective client is still expecting you and make sure you and the prospect have each other's contact details available in case of any last-minute alterations to the meeting.

By confirming on the actual day that the meeting is going ahead, the first step medical interviewer can reduce the likelihood that the prospective client fails to attend the meeting. There are useful resources available online with specific advice on improving attendance at agreed meetings [15, 16].

5. Be Prepared to Undertake More Follow-Up

After meeting a client F2F, planning an aesthetic intervention is typically agreed 40% of the time [17]. This means that, more often than not, there will be no planning conversion during any particular meeting. With this scenario in mind, you should prepare to arrange further follow-up after the initial meeting.

The type of follow-up you offer will depend on what happened in the first meeting. You may choose to telephone the prospect, arrange a further F2F session, book a demonstration or, ideally, arrange a time to sign off on a sale.

Although the exact format will differ, in all cases it is worth preparing an e-mail that summarises the discussion so far for the prospective client. The e-mail should be dispatched no later than 24 h after the meeting. The purpose of this recap e-mail is to consolidate the discussion so far, offer the client a chance to respond with feedback and invite any questions that have since occurred to the prospective client.

Whatever the result of the F2F meeting, remember to express your gratitude for the client's time and interest in the follow-up mail or other communication. This sends the message that you respect the clients and leaves you in a good position to make further contact in the future [2]. They should remember you as polite and helpful.

2.2.5   Fifth Step: Ways to Make the Meeting Effective

With most of the preparation for the meeting now completed, it is time to turn to ways in which you can make the meeting as effective as possible at converting prospective clients into repeat customers. When meeting F2F with prospective clients, there are numerous factors to consider, such as the kind of person you are going to meet, what type of communicative skills are needed, including non-verbal, and the length of time to set for the meeting. When making a sales pitch, it is vital to squeeze the highest possible value out of the time you have available.

2.2.5.1   Talking to C-Level Executives

Virtually all sales representatives aspire to get in contact with the C-level executives in a company. However, once you do manage to achieve this aspiration, it is vital that you do not squander the opportunity by being underprepared.

It is characteristic of C-level executives that they spend a great deal of time attending various meetings. Since such business people have already had considerable experience of sales representatives of different kinds at every stage of their career, they may set a high standard if you wish to impress them and achieve a sale. You must absolutely "sell" the approach you take.

Concentrate in particular on the pain points a client tells you about and focus in on any company objectives that relate to your product or service. A recent IBM document [18] offers the further advice that CEOs are usually more willing to discuss company strategy than to go over the technical details of products or services.

2.2.5.2   Body Language

A key insight to remember in meeting F2F is that a higher percentage of the communicative content comes from body language and extra-verbal cues than from the precise words that you say.

The following are a few of the effective ways to use body language when having F2F meetings:

Hands: Be careful how you shake hands and where you put your hands. A firm, strong handshake conveys the impression that the salesperson has personal strength and confidence in a good product or service. When sitting, the hands should be placed in front of you or to the side and the fingers are kept together, which again conveys a confident approach.

Eye Contact: It is generally a good eye idea to make eye contact with prospective clients for around 50% of the time in the meeting. Do not overdo eye contact, as this can make a prospective client feel uncomfortable. If eye contact falls to too low a level, the impression conveyed is that your heart is not in the sale.

Posture: When standing, keep your back as straight as possible, whilst turning your body in the direction of the prospective client. This posture produces an air of confidence. If you cross your arms, this can put a barrier between you and the client, so it is better to keep the arms in a more neutral position, around the level of the waist.

Once again, there are several useful resources available online to help with the details of body language to use in F2F meetings.

We now turn to an absolutely key aspect of any F2F sales meeting, i.e. the opportunity to actually close on a deal and sign off a sale [2].

2.2.6 Sixth Step: Closing on a Sale

Closing on a sale is the most challenging, but the most satisfying, outcome from a client meeting. It is common, however, for salespeople to finish meetings without having secured agreement on a purchase, and this indecisive conclusion can make subsequent follow-up even harder than the initial meeting.

1. Be Ready from the Start

   The more well-informed you are, the stronger the position you find yourself in. This is especially the case where the meeting occurs F2F. The initial background information you have obtained about the prospective client, coupled with in-depth product knowledge, puts you in a strong position to direct the meeting according to the client's requirements, maximising the chances of it concluding with a sale.

2. Creating a Sense of Urgency in the Client

   It is important to understand how to manipulate a prospective client's emotions and make them feel a decision is an urgent matter, not something to keep delaying indefinitely. Discover where the pain points are and let them see how the pain points are creating problems that your product or service can help to solve. This line of reasoning will usually lead to a sense that a decision needs to be made urgently about the sale, which is exactly the reasoning you wish to encourage.

3. Ask the Client to Decide on the Sale

Due to a fear of being turned down, many sales representatives feel excessively shy about asking the prospective client to sign off on a sale. Yet this is one of the top objectives in an F2F meeting. Provided the meeting has been conducted in an efficient way that leads naturally to the client making a decision about your product or service, there will be no awkwardness about pushing for a decision. Klenty is a sales engagement platform which offers useful advice on the most up-to-date techniques which can help in closing on a sale [19].

4. Efficient Use of Silence

Silence is a valuable way to nudge prospective clients to give an honest account of what their requirements are and where their interests lie. After asking for the client to make a decision about the sale, be prepared to remain waiting in silence for the client to speak. A silence can feel awkward but give space to let clients explain their reasoning. Do not talk yourself out of a sale simply in order to avoid a gap in the conversation [2].

5. Follow-Up

It is a regrettable fact about selling that it often requires multiple meetings before clients agree to buy. Indeed, the average number of meetings needed to lead to a sale is four [19]. If a meeting ends without a decision and follow-up is going to be needed, try to ensure you have an agreement on the timing of the next meeting and what you will discuss on that occasion.

The ability to be patient and act strategically are key factors in achieving sales with the majority of prospective clients. Nonetheless, there are some prospects who represent a greater challenge than the average individual. Even very experienced sales representatives may find themselves encountering prospective clients who act aggressively towards them or seem determined to undermine whatever they have to say. In such circumstances, it may be quite impossible to prevent this type of unwanted behaviour, but there are some actions which can make a meeting of this kind proceed in a more productive fashion. If you face somebody who is especially challenging to deal with, it helps a great deal to realise that such attitudes are probably shown towards other people, too, and it is not your fault that the person is behaving in such an unproductive way. Try to avoid getting too anxious or angry and concentrate on maintaining a positive frame of mind. Do not get sucked into a conflict, although this does not mean letting the person dominate you and make unreasonable demands. Likewise, avoid letting the encounter turn into a dominance competition with that individual.

The most appropriate way to deal with this scenario, in fact, is to remain firm and professional and bring the meeting back towards its intended purpose, which is to establish the pain points the prospective client currently has and the difficulties the firm is currently encountering. Explain why you believe the product or service you are selling has the potential to ease the pain and help overcome the challenges.

If you focus on how you can help the prospect by selling him or her a solution, you will find yourself focusing less on their unappealing or inappropriate behaviour and more on the business of arranging a sale [2].

2.2.7 Seventh Step: Follow-Up Your Clients

As stated earlier, it is not uncommon for an initial meeting to require several follow-up activities before a sale can be finally agreed upon. Unless this follow-up is undertaken in an efficient manner, there is a risk that no sale will ever come out of your effort.

To avoid the danger that either you or your prospective client end up failing to answer each other's calls or e-mails, make sure you arrange suitable follow-up whilst you are in the initial F2F meeting.

2.2.7.1 Create a List of Clear Action Points

Towards the close of your initial meeting, ensure you discuss follow-up with your prospective client. Be clear on what format follow-up will take, whether that be a further F2F meeting, telephone call or a demonstration of the product or service. Set a definite time. It is best to set out clearly exactly what the next steps are and make sure that both you and the prospect agree on what should happen next.

2.2.7.2 Send Your Notes on the Meeting to Your Prospective Client

A brief summary outlining the key points from your initial meeting is a vital part of follow-up. It is worth bearing in mind that the prospective client may also have met other sales representatives and it is important to keep it clear in the client's mind what you spoke about and what makes your product or service special.

There is an informative guide available online, which covers how to compose a suitable follow-up e-mail [20].

2.2.7.3 Be Appreciative

Showing your prospective clients that you value their ideas and the time they put aside for you is important. You can do this by sending a thank you note. If they offered you any advice or guidance, make sure you acknowledge it in your note. After writing a polite and appreciative note of this kind, any subsequent contact will be easier and not perceived as "pushy".

2.2.7.4 Be Solution-Focused

A common error committed by sales representatives is to have too narrow a focus on getting a sale signed off. Instead, as with the initial F2F meeting, pay most attention to how your product or service can make life more comfortable for your clients and solve their business challenges. Offer illustrative business cases or present case studies which reveal the advantages your solution has. Any related articles may also be shared. Aim to offer helpful support and insight, rather than a narrow focus on signing off on a deal.

2.2.7.5   Judge When Follow-Up Is No Longer Appropriate

It has been found that follow-up never goes beyond a single attempt in 44% of sales encounters [21]. However, in 80% of cases, there were a minimum of five follow-up activities before a sale was finally agreed [21].

Whilst it is sometimes necessary to send a final e-mail to a prospective client who no longer responds to your calls or messages, make sure the e-mail expresses your willingness to re-establish contact, if the prospect's situation changes in the future [2].

2.2.7.6   Advice on Presenting F2F for Maximum Effect

When you encounter a particularly impressive presenter, it is worth taking a few moments to analyse what impressed you most about the presentation. Some presenters have the ability to engage you totally in their presentation. But for many people, speaking in public is an anxiety-inducing experience. For these people, it is useful to have some techniques for coping with the stage fright they experience. They may feel reassured by realising many people experience sweaty hands and indigestion when they are about to speak. Remember, too, that speaking at a conference or in front of a group of people is actually a fantastic opportunity to put across vital messages about your product or service and to share success stories and opinions. Speaking well in public can bring significant rewards. Indeed, there is a growing demand for people in leadership positions, such as CEOs, to speak in public. So, however anxious the thought may make you, it is well worth conquering the fear and getting up to speak.

1. *Believe In Yourself:* Because you were chosen to speak, surely that means you have some expertise on a topic, or at least others think that about you?
2. *Know About Your Listeners:* Consider carefully who the members of the audience will be, why they are there and what they may want to learn from your presentation. If the speech is at a conference, you can ask for a list of likely attendees in advance, to help you prepare.
3. *Consider the Topic:* What is it about the topic that is of current relevance and interest? One possible technique is to think about some problem related to the topic and then frame the presentation as a solution to that issue, perhaps through an illustrative case study. The presentation can then move onto more general aspects of the topic.
4. *Decide on the Take Home Message from the Presentation:* It is often useful to mention the key messages three times—tell the audience what the message will be, tell them the message, then tell them what message you told them.
5. *Stay Within the Time Limits:* Avoid at all costs the temptation to pad out a presentation to make it longer.
6. *Add Visual Interest:* Make use of presentation software (such as PowerPoint or Impress) or give out illustrated notes. The use of visual props also adds interest.
7. *Tell a Story:* Use storytelling techniques to spin a tale that keeps your audience engaged by relating the topic to everyday life. A case study can also fit this format.

8. ***Be Who You Are:*** Authenticity in speaking comes across very sympathetically to audiences.
9. ***Get the Audience to Participate:*** Encourage interactivity by throwing out questions, doing quick polls or asking the audience members to interact with the person sitting next to them.
10. ***Challenge the Audience to Act on Your Message:*** As you conclude your presentation, ensure you challenge the listeners to act on your message. When they act on your recommendation, they will keep remembering your presentation.

An F2F presentation is something that deserves your best efforts. You owe it to yourself and to the audience to prepare yourself thoroughly before you present. It is the preparation stage that makes the difference between a barely adequate and an excellent presentation. If you are adequately prepared, there is no particular reason to feel anxious about presenting [22].

2.3 Factors That Make F2F Presentations More Convincing Than Other Formats

As the possibilities for presentations to be delivered virtually increase and the technology allows for greater audience interactivity and engagement with the topic, it is inevitable that F2F presentation will be seen as a valuable resource which must not be squandered. Since F2F involves a greater investment in time and money for travel than online formats, there is a corresponding increase in the expectations from the format.

Indeed, it is reasonable to question the extent to which F2F can continue to exist, when there are such obvious economic benefits to online presentations. However, F2F presentations do still have an edge thanks to a number of unique features, as we will now discuss.

In the first place, presentations delivered F2F are typically more convincing than remotely delivered presentations. It is a common experience that if you really want to convince someone to do something, you go and see that individual in-person. Likewise, speaking on the telephone is usually more effective in getting someone to act than asking in an e-mail.

There are six factors that help to influence someone to act, as identified by Robert Cialdini, in his well-known work, "The Psychology of Persuasion". These factors are as follows:

Reciprocity. The tendency to repay a good turn
When individuals present F2F, it is usually apparent they have made particular effort to get ready and come to a specific venue to speak. This means that audiences already feel more obliged to listen to their words. It is far easier to abandon an online session that appears uninteresting than to leave an F2F presentation. Leaving an F2F presentation causes a much guiltier feeling than logging out from a Zoom meeting, for example.

Showing you are committed and consistent. When people commit to an idea, they prefer not to back out

Attendance at an F2F presentation, which requires giving up time to be present, indicates a degree of commitment. According to this line of reasoning, there is an increased likelihood that people who attend a presentation in-person will be influenced by what they hear.

Social proof: Others' reactions guide our own reaction

When sitting as members of an audience, individuals' reactions to a presentation are guided by how other audience members are behaving. This is not the case when the same presentation is viewed, for example, in the privacy of an individual's own home. This effect is termed "social proof".

The influence of authority

People who are viewed as authority figures attract more obedience than the average person. A presenter in an F2F event appears as the authority on a subject.

Liking people makes us trust them more

Whereas impressions about an individual met virtually usually take some time to form, the F2F format encourages people to make rapid judgements on whether they like the presenter. These first impressions count, as a favourable first impression makes the presenter seem more credible.

Scarcity of any resource raises its value

It is a relatively unusual experience to attend an F2F presentation. The scarcity of such opportunities gives it an air of exclusivity. By contrast, clicking on a video presentation on a platform such as YouTube or Dailymotion does not seem like accessing a scarce resource, and it is accordingly less valued.

To take a specific example. There are many educational and informative presentations by acknowledged experts hosted by the TED organisation. Even though these events are also available for free on the web, with high production qualities evident in the filming, there is still a large number of people willing to travel and pay to attend in-person.

Human psychology evolved long before remote communication was possible and there are special adaptations that favour F2F meetings. It seems unlikely that F2F will one day fail to offer an advantage in terms of persuasiveness and impact [23].

2.4   Ways to Become More Skilled at F2F Communication

At its most fundamental, communication is simply the act of passing a message from one person to one or several others. This apparent simplicity is somewhat deceptive, however. There are multiple ways in which communication can fail. It is common to misunderstand other people or to be misunderstood yourself. Indeed, communicative failure occurs much more frequently than is commonly realised.

Although there are numerous ways in which communication can fail, there are also ways in which it is possible to become more effective in communicating. There are undoubted advantages to improving F2F communication, but the techniques involved generally require some practice until the benefits become apparent. The following sections describe actions presenters can take to improve their F2F communication skills [24].

2.4.1 Pay Attention to Your Posture

Communication may seem to be primarily verbal, but there are many non-verbal elements that contribute to meaning, including posture. For F2F presentations, the ideal posture appears relaxed and open. Whether sitting or standing, keep your back straight and turn towards the audience. This posture signals approachability, which will make the audience more willing to listen to your ideas. If the posture is not upright and you tend to slouch, the audience will be less attentive. Conversely, arms crossed across the chest sends the message that you are closed and even hostile to your audience. Pay attention to negative body language, as this sends signals that interfere with your intended message and make communication less efficient.

2.4.2 Preserve Eye Contact

A great deal of attention is paid to eye contact when training speakers. This emphasis is certainly warranted as eye contact conveys very effectively that you respect your audience. Furthermore, eye contact indicates that you are sincere, that you believe what you are saying and can be trusted. It also hints at a degree of vulnerability, which makes the speaker appear more likeable. Thus, attending to eye contact is a key element in F2F communication generally.

Some people find it a little disconcerting to maintain a high degree of eye contact. If this is the case, you can look at a point just beyond where the other person's eyes are. This then appears to the other person as normal eye contact. Avoid staring at the ground, as this conveys a negative impression. Conversely, judge carefully how much eye contact to maintain. You do not want other people to feel you are staring at them, as this is an uncomfortable sensation.

2.4.3 Select Carefully the Words to Use

Given the central importance of words to convey your ideas, it is clearly necessary to select the language you use with appropriate consideration. Aim for a language register (level) that is appropriate to the audience. For example, a speech to a general or mixed audience should avoid technical words, the meaning of which may be unfamiliar and which will then become a distraction. However, if you are addressing fellow experts, the language should be as precise as possible, which will entail use of technical vocabulary. If you are presenting to children, bear in mind that they have a smaller vocabulary than adults and try to convey the message in a simpler way, although work hard to avoid the danger of patronising your audience.

2.4.4   Ensure You Can Be Heard

Being audible is vital to effective communication. If the audience is missing some words, they may misconstrue what you are saying or fail to understand at all. Speak at a volume where audiences can hear without straining to do so. If there are more than a handful of listeners, a microphone becomes a very valuable aid. Check in all cases that you are being properly heard.

Nonetheless, you should also pay attention not to come across as too loud. In such a case, you may seem to be shouting at the audience, which makes you appear aggressive and hostile. It can also irritate the audience if the microphone amplifies the noise excessively. The optimal level is the one where the message is getting efficiently delivered without interference.

In virtual presentations, there is the analogous issue of poor transmitted sound quality. A number of technical solutions to improving the sound are on the market, such as ezTalks. Use of high definition video and sound helps to make the presentation clearer.

2.4.5   Remember to Listen

Communication is not unidirectional. When presenting, you want the audience to receive your message, but this does not entail ignoring messages the audience sends you. Leave pauses in the presentation, invite feedback and think carefully how to respond. Try to empathise with the audience. Being an empathic listener is a highly valuable communication skill that all presenters should acquire [24].

References

1. 3.5 face-to-face communication. Part 3: the medium. https://pressbooks.bccampus.ca/mission-messagemedium/chapter/3-5-face-to-face-communication/. Accessed 3 Oct 2021.
2. 7 Steps to effective face-to-face meetings. https://managementevents.com/insights/sales/7-steps-to-effective-face-to-face-meetings/. Accessed 3 Oct 2021.
3. How to lead online meetings: no hiding and practical tips. https://mgrush.com/blog/online-meetings/. Accessed 13 Oct 2021.
4. 15 Surprising stats on networking and face-to-face communication. https://blog.hubspot.com/sales/face-to-face-networking-stats?__hstc=63639152.72d49eb70daa874804aeca02b9680831.1633293209898.1633293209898.1633293209898.1&__hssc=63639152.2.1633293209899&__hsfp=3926047488.
5. By every measure, face-to-face meetings beat virtual meetings. https://www.themeeting-magazines.com/cit/every-measure-face-face-meetings-beat-virtual-meetings/. Accessed 13 Oct 2021.
6. How to optimize online networking. https://managementevents.com/news/how-to-optimize-virtual-networking/?utm_source=me_website&utm_medium=pillar_page&utm_campaign=face_to_face&utm_term=redirectME&utm_content=marketing. Accessed 13 Oct 2021.
7. What is warm calling? https://www.thebalancecareers.com/what-is-warm-calling-2917380. Accessed 14 Oct 2021.

8. The Sales Hunter. https://thesaleshunter.com. Accessed 14 Oct 2021.
9. The impact of social selling. https://www.slideshare.net/linkedin-sales-solutions/the-impact-of-social-selling-on-sales-perception-45184696. Accessed 14 Oct 2021.
10. 6 Strategies to get more sales meetings with prospects. https://www.calendar.com/blog/get-more-sales-meetings-with-prospects/. Accessed 14 Oct 2021.
11. 130 Eye-opening sales statistics. https://spotio.com/blog/sales-statistics/. Accessed 14 Oct 2021.
12. Social buying meets social selling: how trusted networks improve the purchase experience. https://business.linkedin.com/content/dam/business/sales-solutions/global/en_US/c/pdfs/idc-wp-247829.pdf. Accessed 14 Oct 2021.
13. The surprising reality of how many emails are sent per day in 2021. https://techjury.net/blog/how-many-emails-are-sent-per-day/. Accessed 14 Oct 2021.
14. How to get appointments with decision makers. https://managementevents.com/news/how-to-get-appointments-with-decision-makers/. Accessed 14 Oct 2021.
15. Sales appointments: getting prospects to show up. https://www.salesbuzz.com/sales-appointments-getting-prospects-to-show-up/. Accessed 16 Oct 2021.
16. 20 highly-effective sales prospecting techniques for 2021. https://www.yesware.com/blog/sales-prospecting-techniques/. Accessed 16 Oct 2021.
17. The return on investment of U.S. business travel. https://www.oxfordeconomics.com/Media/Default/Industry%20verticals/Tourism/US%20Travel%20Association-%20ROI%20on%20US.%20Business%20Travel.pdf. Accessed 16 Oct 2021.
18. Calling on the CEO - executive relationship marketing. https://www-2000.ibm.com/partner-world/industries/pdfs/Calling_on_the_CEO.pdf. Accessed 16 Oct 2021.
19. 20 Modern sales closing techniques that will help you win more deals. https://blog.klenty.com/sales-closing-techniques/. Accessed 16 Oct 2021.
20. A complete guide to sales follow-up. https://keap.com/business-success-blog/sales/sales-process/sales-follow-up-techniques. Accessed 17 Oct 2021.
21. How often to follow up on sales leads? https://www.salesmate.io/blog/how-often-to-follow-up-on-sales-leads/. Accessed 17 Oct 2021.
22. 10 Tips for powerful face to face presentations. 7 Aug 2017. http://www.ruralscope.com.au/Blog/ArtMID/3132/ArticleID/537814/10-Tips-for-Powerful-Face-to-Face-Presentations. Accessed 3 Oct 2021.
23. Mitchell O. The 6 reasons why face-to-face presenting is more persuasive. https://speaking-aboutpresenting.com/presentation-philosophy/6-reasons-face-to-face-presenting-persuasive/. Accessed 3 Oct 2021.
24. How to improve face to face communication skills. https://eztalks.com/unified-communications/how-to-improve-face-to-face-communication-skills.html. Accessed 3 Oct 2021.

3.1 Using Technology Whilst Presenting

There is a plethora of technological innovations available to assist with presentations. This chapter addresses the ways that technology can contribute towards impactful presentations. A distinction will also be drawn between using technology in face-to-face (F2F) presentations and using it when delivering online.

The chapter will also consider how a hypothetical sales manager, Lara, with responsibility for a global portfolio, can make the best use of technology to increase sales. Lara is a sales executive working for a major laboratory equipment manufacturer. This will help to show how solutions can be applied in real life.

We also discuss the theoretical aspects of the topic. Technology, when used creatively and thoughtfully, enables individuals to reach a far wider range of prospective clients than would otherwise be the case.

In discussing a particular technology, we will consider how a business person with an international portfolio can become more productive through its use [1].

3.1.1 PowerPoint and Its Equivalents

For F2F presentations, PowerPoint is effectively the standard application to use. There are a number of equivalents, however, such as the open source tool, Impress. This type of application allows the user to generate attractive slides combining graphics, spreadsheet functionality, links, animations and more. This software is reliable, standard and the learning curve is not too steep. In experienced hands, very creative effects can be achieved. However, the default slide design consists of lists of information, and this may not be the optimal way to present a topic to an audience. Whilst PowerPoint can be used collaboratively, some other solutions are better for this purpose. When presenting F2F in this way, some form of screen or projector needs to be available, which may not always be the case.

© The Author(s), under exclusive license to Springer Nature
Switzerland AG 2023
C. C. Cingi et al., *Improving Online Presentations*,
https://doi.org/10.1007/978-3-031-28328-4_3

Lara might benefit from having a standard slide deck that can be used when presenting to prospective clients that she can drive to. She may like to send this standard slide deck to prospects at an early stage to introduce her product portfolio.

3.1.2   Google Slides

Another possible application for generating a set of slides is Google Slides, which is part of the Google Docs package of web-based software. This application benefits from being extremely straightforward to learn and is set up to easily permit remote collaboration. Unsurprisingly, perhaps, it lacks many of the high level features of a program such as PowerPoint or Impress, but it is suitable if the slides are mainly of a functional type and a high level of aesthetic appeal is unnecessary. There are several templates that the user can access to assemble a slide set quickly and easily.

The Google Docs suite is very suitable for online collaboration, which can be done in real time. Sharing any documents you generate is also straightforward. Thus, teams that need to collaborate may like this solution. Lara could use it to get feedback or ideas from clients or when she needs to work with colleagues to produce a presentation [1].

3.1.3   Video Software

There are a number of software applications which can convert between video formats (including the capability of digitising older video from analogue sources), which then means that a film can be embedded in a presentation. In this way, it is possible for Lara to show a product demonstration video from within her presentation, without the need to open a second application to do so.

Video is a good way to introduce variety and interest into a presentation. It is eye-catching and a good counterpoint to slides containing text. If a company has older promotional video materials captured in VHS format, for example, these can be converted into a digital format and then edited, to provide short clips, for example. Examples of video editing software include the proprietary Windows Movie Maker and Adobe Premier Pro, or the open source OpenShot.

A further way to use video editing software is to add notes to a video which help to emphasise a particular point. Lara might wish to annotate a video to show how a design feature of particular equipment helps to solve a client's particular issues.

3.1.4   Screen Casting

Screen captures are videos which show the appearance on a person's screen as they are using a particular piece of software or carrying out a particular task. The capture allows movement of the mouse, cursor position and any cascading menus to be seen. This may be preferable to a simple textual description of how to do the task. It allows software features to be readily demonstrated [1].

Since Lara's portfolio includes the software needed to run the laboratory equipment, a screen capture would be very helpful to highlight how easy the software is to use. It would be more effective and engaging than listing the steps in order.

3.2   Advice on How to Deliver an Excellent Online Presentation

Online presentations used in business fulfil a variety of functions, including giving information, outlining a proposal or showcasing innovative products or services. Presentations are usually in the form of a teleconference or video call. They may be intended for a variety of different audiences [2].

3.2.1   Make a Powerful Start

It is sometimes said that online presentations resemble a trip on an aeroplane, insofar as the audience (passengers) are most alert during take-off and landing, but otherwise find the experience not especially interesting. The point of the analogy is to stress the importance of beginning well, since that is when you audience will be at their most alert and receptive.

The start of a presentation is the time when you establish the tone of what is to follow. It is essential to make a positive initial impression if you want the audience to have trust in you and feel comfortable. A strong beginning energises the audience for the body of the presentation, where most of the key messages and evidence will be found. A lacklustre start means you will struggle enormously to energise the audience for the rest of your presentation.

What that means in practical terms is that, whenever you present online, you need to do so without making awkward mistakes and in as smooth a fashion as you can. How to achieve this is by paying attention to the ways in which presentations tend to get derailed in the vital first few minutes.

Make sure the computer is properly set up, with no compatibility issues between the various components, such as the sound, video and network connection. Perform updates well in advance of the presentation and test all the equipment first. If there are computer-related problems at the start of the presentation, this can unfortunately make the presenter appear unprepared, or even incompetent.

Ensure No Distractions Occur Turn your mobile phone to silent mode, disable any desktop notifications, switch off any noisy equipment, such as air conditioning, and keep children or pets out of the room from which you are presenting. Since background noise tends to be amplified through headphones, you need to be especially careful about this issue when presenting online.

Wear a Suitable Outfit to Present   Just because a presentation will be online, it does not mean that the presenter should dress down. Dress with similar care to how you would for an F2F presentation. Do not assume that you do not need to wear a pair of trousers, because you will remain seated throughout. It is better to be slightly over-smart than to appear scruffy. You will need to wear an outfit that stands out from the background, although very flamboyant colours may be a bad idea, since they may distract your audience.

Remain Upbeat   The emotional state of the presenter is revealed in a number of ways, including the tone of voice presenters use. Avoid giving the impression you are tense, angry or anxious. If you find yourself feeling that way before you present, try to unwind a little before you start. If you sound upbeat and full of confidence, the presentation will have a much more positive impact [2].

3.2.2   Remember the Mnemonic: $I^2S^2A^2Q^2$

This mnemonic reminds you of the key features to include in a presentation for maximum positive impact. There are two items beginning with "I", two with "s", two with "a" and two with "q".

Break the **ice** first. It is a good idea to have one or two icebreaker activities available to use before you start your presentation proper. There are several types of icebreakers that are suitable for use in online presentations.

Illustrate what you say. Get your audience to engage their senses by recalling a previous incident or describe in detail a scene that you want them to imagine.

Tell **stories** as you go. Anecdotes featuring yourself or someone else are useful in getting the audience's attention, provided the story is relatively succinct and has a good punchline.

Surprising statistics make the audience sit up and question their previous assumptions.

Aphorisms are proverbs or sayings that everybody has heard of. The trick is to work the saying into the presentation. One way to enhance the effect is to turn the aphorism around in some way relevant to the presentation. Lara, for example, could write a pun into the software presentation by saying something like "a switch in time saves F9" in place of the more familiar "a stitch in time saves nine".

Analogy helps make the meaning clearer. By comparing a product to a more familiar item, for example, you can make the unfamiliar topic seem less daunting. Lara could compare cytometry equipment to the part of a vending machine that distinguishes between different coins, for example.

Questions can make your audience engage with the presentation. Challenge your audience to think themselves about an issue, or use rhetorical questions, which you then answer.

Quotations are very suitable for the start of a presentation. However, any quotation should be both clearly relevant to what follows and from a respected source.

3.2.3   Make the Ending Memorable

By the time your presentation reaches the end, you are hoping that the audience will have been able to learn something of value and feel motivated to take a new action. Having reached this stage successfully, it is vital not to end in a way that undermines your achievement up to now. The ending is just as much a part of the presentation as the beginning and main body. The following sections highlight ways to end a presentation on a high note.

Offer a Straightforward Answer to End the Presentation Avoid loading your final slides with too much information. The main body of the presentation is where the main information belongs. At the last stage of the presentation, the audience has the right to expect a persuasive, easily digested message about the topic.

Make It Clear the Presentation Is Ending There should be a slide that signals you have reached the end of the presentation, by reiterating the "take home message". The take home message may be a succinct summary of the information provided or a call for the audience to take some particular action. Do not let the presentation peter out with a weak-sounding comment such as "that's about it, unless you have anything to ask?"

Give the Audience Something to Take Away from the Presentation Audiences love receiving a small gift at the end of an F2F presentation, such as a copy of a paper. This practice can be adapted for online presentations, where you can send the audience a downloadable document, such as a summary report or a paper of relevance to the subject. PDF format is especially suitable for these kinds of giveaways, as they are then easy to print out if required.

Invite the Audience to Take Action on a Topic When you want an audience to take a particular action, an emotional appeal works better than one grounded purely on rational choice. If purchasing a product or service will solve a particular pain point for businesses, emphasise the peace of mind that comes with the solution, rather than stating that it reduces the problem by 38.9% in 81% of cases. If you are selling internet security products, for instance, emphasise the dire consequences of being unprepared for a cyberattack, both personally and as a firm, then reassure your prospective clients that your security product will make such nightmares highly unlikely to affect you. Emphasise how the client can focus on the good things, rather than dealing with problems all the time.

Have a humorous twist to end the presentation. Humour has the potential to impact audiences in a deep and enduring way. There are a number of techniques which can introduce humour into a presentation, some of which are used by stand-up comedians or other comedy writers. An essential element in humour is surprise. You might ask the audience a question early on in your presentation, and then answer it at the end in an unexpected (and humorous) way. Alternatively, you could begin a story, then wait to tell the conclusion at the end of the presentation. This is a similar technique to one used by the late Ronnie Corbett in his show, "The Two Ronnies". He would introduce a tall story, then not give the punchline until right at the end, having digressed meanwhile onto several other topics.

3.2.4   Let Your Face Be Seen

Human beings have an innate fascination with faces that appears early on in development and persists throughout life. A 1963 study by Robert L Fantz demonstrated a clear preference in infants for gazing at faces, rather than other objects. This finding has since been replicated many times. Presenters can take advantage of this preference for looking at faces by ensuring their face appears on the screen at the same time as any slides. Most online presentation factors allow the presenter to set up the screen so the presenter's face remains visible. This is a straightforward way to make you seem more relatable and likeable.

To take even greater advantage of this preference for audiences seeing the presenter, you might move back from the webcam or set up a camera at an angle to catch sight of your whole face, arms and torso. This then allows the audience to observe hand gestures, which are a key component in creating presence. It has been noted by researchers that the greatest proportion of overall meaning is actually conveyed by body language, of which hand gestures are a part. Therefore, setting the camera up to show more of you is a definite advantage in terms of both presence and conveying meaning.

There are several ways to use your hands to improve presentation delivery, including the following:

- Wave hello to the audience, which establishes you are friendly
- Gesture with your hands when explaining a point
- Make sure your hands are visible whilst you listen to questions [2]

3.2.5   Presenting from a Standing Position Is Best

It is wrong to assume that you have to be seated to deliver an online presentation. In fact, there are several advantages to standing, rather than sitting, when presenting.

Firstly, standing up allows you to breathe to the maximum possible extent. This gives your voice more power and makes you sound more confident. Not only is the sound deeper and louder when standing, you can also convey more variety in your tone of voice. The posture when standing also makes the presenter appear more self-assured, as long as the chest is held up and the back kept straight.

Wherever possible, use a lectern or tall table, where you can place your laptop or tablet. If there is no other suitable furniture available, a kitchen worktop may be at nearly the right level. However, if there is no alternative but to sit throughout the presentation, at least ensure you remain sitting firmly upright throughout [2].

3.2.6   Provide a Bonus Near the Start

If your presentation includes a particularly useful tip or suggestion, it is more advantageous to offer it at an early stage in the presentation than to wait until the end. Receiving a gift of this kind will act as a great motivator for the audience to keep attentive for the rest of the presentation [2].

3.2.7   Make the Best Use of Visual Aids

Visual aids are a component of a great presentation and can serve various purposes, such as:

- Keeping the audience's attention
- Making information more memorable
- Reducing complex information to a more readily intelligible form
- Providing greater variety in slide appearance

It is therefore advisable to add some visual interest to whatever topic you are presenting on. There are many distractions for audiences listening to an online presentation and thus retaining the audience's focus is challenging. Any way you can improve this focus is beneficial, since a lack of focus from an audience member greatly reduces the chances they will remember your message. According to researchers [3], 3 days after presentation, 10% recall occurred for information that was given in textual form only, whereas 65% recall was possible when the information was paired with a suitable illustration. Thus, it is clear that adding a visual element to a presentation is a straightforward way to enhance retention of the message.

The following are some ideas for the kind of visual elements that add variety to a text-based presentation:

- Photos licensed from stock collections
- Videos from sites such as YouTube or Dailymotion
- Bar graphs
- Pie charts
- Animated images (i.e. GIFs)
- Internet memes
- Cartoon drawings
- Other types of art, such as digital paintings

Adding visual elements is a simple tactic to "spice up" otherwise dry material, but only when done in a carefully considered way. Whilst visuals always add variety, there are some ways in which they may actually detract from the message you want to give, such as in the following scenarios:

When the illustration does not match the point you are trying to make. If Lara wants to emphasise the need to calibrate the equipment on a daily basis but illustrates this with a cartoon of a dog playing with a ball, her clients may laugh but miss the point.
Inappropriate illustrations for an audience may confuse the message. A pie chart may be too simplistic for an audience of PhD scientists, but too hard to understand for an audience of primary school children.
Distracting materials can direct the audience onto the wrong topic.
Visuals that do not simplify and organise information are not helpful.
When using a video, make sure it is trimmed to the right length.

Where any of these scenarios applies, the simple rule is to rethink the need for the visual. If you decide to keep it, make sure it is relevant and informative, not merely decorative [2]. It is a good discipline when preparing a slide set to write down the rationale for each visual. Not only does this practice help to ensure only valuable visuals are added, it also helps when you present as you may need to introduce the visual and explain what it illustrates.

3.2.8 Introduce Interactive Elements

One of the key disadvantages to presenting online is that keeping an audience engaged on the topic is even harder than in an F2F presentation. As well as attractive, relevant and informative visual elements, another key way to make the presentation better is by making it interactive [2].

3.2.9 Use of Props

The use of visual props can greatly enhance the audience's interest in what you are saying.
So, what are the ways to introduce visual props into virtual presentations? First of all, props should be used for a specific purpose, such as explaining a complicated subject, showing what a product actually looks like, for humorous effect, or to make the presentation more memorable. It goes without saying that a prop should not be used if it will distract from the message of the presentation. Likewise, a prop must be something the audience will actually be able to see.
Accordingly, a very small, difficult-to-see prop might not be suitable for a video call. To show the prop, it may be necessary to briefly halt the presentation and make the video full screen, so that the whole object can be seen.
One useful piece of advice about using a prop is not to reveal the prop until you show it completely. If the audience catches a tantalising glimpse of the prop, but cannot see it properly, their minds will be on the prop rather than on what you are saying [2].

3.2.10 Introduce a Quiz or Poll into Your Presentation

Another exciting way to make a presentation more appealing is by introducing a quiz, survey or poll. Lara could, for example, ask her prospective clients for their opinions about a certain type of equipment before then providing some facts. The audience enjoys seeing what everybody thinks and discovering if they themselves were right or wrong.

Some details on applications that can be used for online quizzes and polls are outlined below [2].

3.2.11 Real-Time Questions and Answers

The introduction of live Q and A's into an online presentation is an effective way to increase the level of interactivity.

Suppose that Lara was presenting to a group of her peers about the best ways to overcome objections to the purchase of more up-to-date laboratory equipment. She might throw out the question, "What types of objections do you come across when you recommend upgrading existing equipment?" This should allow her to elicit a variety of objections heard by salespeople. The next step is what makes this exercise really valuable for engaging the audience. She then opens the next slide, which contains suggested answers to the objections elicited. This way of presenting means that the presentation has acquired a newly enhanced relevance for her peers, as it is answering the very problems they have described. Thus the interactivity, combined with a smooth transition to possible solutions, will increase audience engagement [2].

3.2.12 Shorten Your Presentation

Be careful that you do not end up repeating yourself in a presentation, as this will definitely bore your audience. This kind of repetition or padding can creep in from various sources, such as adding extra information that is not strictly relevant to the topic, giving supplementary evidence to support a point that you have already established, including visuals that add nothing extra to the topic, or wordy explanations (prolixity).

Presenters need to aim for the presentation to be as concise as possible, but without omitting any information needed to fully understand the topic. Having a few key points written down on cue cards is a practical way to keep the word count down whilst still covering the essential material adequately.

As with an F2F presentation, an online presentation should aim for simplicity and being readily understandable. Remember that watching an online presentation may be quite tiring for audiences, especially if they are watching on a small screen on a mobile device, for example. Eye strain is something that distinguishes online from F2F presentations [2].

3.2.13 Make a Screen Recording When You Practise Presenting

One advantage of delivering a presentation online is that it is possible to practise delivery in very similar circumstances to those of the actual presentation. Usually, you can practise in the room from which you will present, with the same illumination, same computer and software. Practise before you deliver the presentation for real and remember to make a screen recording. In many cases, there is no need to install extra software to achieve this as the functionality already exists on many systems running Windows or the Mac OS.

When the recording is complete, watch it from a critical perspective, asking yourself questions, such as:

- Am I using an appropriate level of hand gestures?
- Is the body language natural-looking, or does it seem awkward?
- Is the sound level clear and is my voice confident-sounding?
- What technical problems did I encounter?
- Does the presentation fit comfortably in the allocated time slot? Not too lengthy or too brief?

You might also benefit from showing the presentation to someone whose feedback you trust, to get a second opinion.

3.2.14 Select the Right Software to Help You

There is an abundance of software applications available to help with online presenting. Choosing the best tool is a vital part of the preparation. Some of the tasks software can help with include:

- Creating new animations
- Designing infographics
- Conference scheduling
- Laying out mind maps
- Selecting suitable illustrations
- Putting the whole presentation together

Whatever the particular requirements of your presentation, the most appropriate tool or tools need to be identified first. It is generally a good idea to utilise one application to put together an interesting slide set and then use different software to find or produce appropriate visuals. The following are a selection of the many currently available applications to help with the task:

3.2.14.1 Pixabay

Adding some visual elements to the text makes the presentation more varied and interesting. Pixabay lets you select, free of charge, videos or images for use in a presentation. There are several million categorised visual assets to choose from, all of a high quality.

3.2.14.2   Canva

Canva is another free option, which offers assistance with all aspects of designing your slide set, with infographics, logo designs, images and templates for your presentation. These elements can be extensively customised. Another notable feature of Canva is the choice of virtual backgrounds, which you can set to appear behind you when presenting with Zoom.

3.2.14.3   Poll Everywhere

Poll Everywhere is an application that allows the user to set up polls or quizzes in real time. These may involve MCQs, choice of true/false, short answers and more. The software works on a variety of devices, including laptops, tablets and mobile telephones. Not only is it straightforward to use, it also offers easy integration with some other software, such as PowerPoint.

3.2.14.4   Krisp

Krisp is a type of noise and echo cancellation software that helps to make the presenter's voice much clearer. It is helpful if you do not have a soundproof room from which to present. It is available both as a standalone application and as a web browser extension. Currently there is the option to use the application for up to 2 h a week free of charge. This software is a real help when presenting from a noisy home or office.

3.2.14.5   PowerPoint, Impress and Keynote

PowerPoint, Impress and Keynote are all applications which are intended to allow you to put together an attractive slide deck, including text, graphics and so forth. Keynote comes as part of the bundled software on Apple systems. PowerPoint is proprietary software created by Microsoft. Impress is part of the OpenOffice and LibreOffice open source office suites and is completely free of charge.

3.2.15 Manage Your Fear of Speaking in Public

For many people, especially if they are not naturally extroverted, the thought of speaking in public can be daunting, terrifying even. In some ways, this fear is no less than if someone were to do an adrenaline sport, such as bungee jumping, for the first time.

In fact, some speakers, however, often they practise public speaking, will always experience some degree of stage fright when called on to speak. In such people, managing that fear is a better option than trying to banish it altogether.

Typically, the fear of public speaking, or stage fright, actually improves over time as you become more experienced at public speaking. Each time a presentation goes well, you tend to feel more confident for the next time you need to present. In time, the fear may be replaced by a positive sense of achievement when you overcome that fear. There are few things as satisfying as having just delivered a presentation that excited and inspired your audience. Each time you present, you will move closer and closer to the ideal presentation [2].

References

1. Lombardo J. Using technology to deliver a presentation: pros, Cons & Strategies. Updated: 08/11/2020.   https://study.com/academy/lesson/using-technology-to-deliver-a-presentation-pros-cons-strategies.html. Accessed 3 Oct 2021.
2. 12 tips to give an amazing online presentation. https://www.scienceofpeople.com/online-presentation/. Accessed 3 Oct 2021.
3. Medina J. Brain rules: 12 principles for surviving and thriving at work, home, and school. Pear Press; 2008.

The Online Presenting Environment, the Equipment to Use and the Materials to Benefit From

4

4.1 Introduction

The content of your presentation and the way you present have always been vital to how successful any presentation is, and this is just as true with online presentations. It is unfortunately not difficult for most people to recall an online presentation where things went horribly wrong, whether because the presenter was inaudible, the presenter disappeared into the background or a baby could be heard crying throughout. In such circumstances, it is no wonder that people only half-listen to the presentation and prefer to do something else instead, like catching up on e-mails. Conversely, there are presentations online that are both highly impactful and technically superb. The difference is not simply a matter of chance. It comes down to foresight and planning. These presenters have wisely chosen the best equipment for the task and set up the presenting environment to facilitate excellence in delivery. The need to acquire the knowledge of creating the best environment to present has never been more pressing, as the drive to virtual delivery, accelerated so much by the recent COVID-19 pandemic, shows no signs of slowing. Thus, more and more individuals find themselves called on to present virtually. If you want to deliver a technically superior presentation, do not wait until the last minute to set up the environment and practise with the equipment. Instead, plan well in advance, so that you can present comfortably, knowing the environment will support you, rather than leave you floundering, as you try to figure out the settings for the webcam [1].

4.2 Setup, Equipment and Materials

The specific setup needed, as well as the equipment to use and materials to choose, differs according to individual requirements. However, there are certain core items that are of particular value to the majority of presenters, who want to present in a professionally competent way from their home office [1].

© The Author(s), under exclusive license to Springer Nature Switzerland AG 2023
C. C. Cingi et al., *Improving Online Presentations*,
https://doi.org/10.1007/978-3-031-28328-4_4

4.2.1   External Webcams

In many cases, presenters rely on the webcam built into their laptops to provide a video feed. However, having an external webcam does offer the opportunity to improve video quality significantly and is much more flexible than the built-in webcam. It is really a question of whether you are aiming for the best quality video or will be satisfied with the basic video available by default. One external webcam that has recently enjoyed significant popularity is the Logitech C920 webcam, which has been well reviewed by both speakers and audiovisual technical experts. However, the high demand for this product has driven up prices, so it may be worth looking at alternative options. The camera should then be set up in such a way that your eyes are at the level of a third of the way down the screen.

Experts also recommend mounting an external camera on the lectern if you aim to stand during your presentation. A tripod may be helpful, although many presenters have found that some ingenuity and experimentation may save a great deal of money. If you can securely mount the camera on a pile of books or something similar, there may be no need to invest in special equipment [1]. It is also worth noting that some digital cameras can also be set up to act as a high quality webcam.

4.2.2   Additional Illumination

Having adequate illumination for your face is of vital importance, since a face in darkness is very hard to make out. This may be especially problematic if your skin tone is already dark. Setting up adequate illumination is not always straightforward, especially with the ordinary lamps that people typically have in their homes or offices. Ring lights offer an effective solution and are used by many virtual presenters, but they may sometimes produce glare when reflected off the presenter's spectacles. Therefore taking precautions is advisable when using them [2]. As well as ring lights, other options include LED panels or softbox lighting kits. The latter equipment, however, can be fairly bulky and may not fit into the space you have available for delivering your presentation [1].

4.2.3   External Microphone

There are few things as guaranteed to ruin an online presentation as having poor audio quality. Conversely, if presenters want to get the maximum attention from their audiences, they need to make sure the audio signal is as clear as possible. There are several ways to achieve this. One option is to use a USB external microphone. A popular choice currently is the Blue Yeti range, although there are many alternatives, which are reviewed online. Another popular choice is the Blue Snowball model. For presenters who intend to stand during their presentations, it may be most practical to use a lapel microphone (lavalier microphone), since this moves as the presenter does, ensuring the audio signal remains clear [1].

4.2.4   Simple, Uncluttered Background

In the majority of cases, ensuring you have a simple, uncluttered background behind you when you present does not call for any extra expenditure. Videoconferencing applications, like Zoom, offer virtual backgrounds, but these add to bandwidth. Two popular choices for a real background are a solid, plain wall or the appearance of a study or library. Whilst it is reasonable to use the natural background of your home if this shows your individual character, it is important to make sure there is nothing on display that should normally be hidden from public view. The background should not distract from the audience's focus on you, the presenter. Getting the audience to focus on an online presentation already presents a challenge. To check there are no distractions, it is worth recording yourself a few times to see if anything unexpectedly catches the eye. In addition to visual distractions, it is important to ensure that there are no distracting sounds, either. Put your phone in silent mode, disable any desktop alerts and make sure no-one will be talking in the background.

Besides the external webcam, microphone, special lighting and appropriate background setup, there are a number of other items which presenters may wish to consider, although they are less essential to the presentation. Examples are a remote slide advancer, teleprompt equipment, a better quality router and possibly an ethernet cable that stretches far enough that you do not need to rely on Wi-Fi. However, these items are more desirable extras than essential core equipment, and it may be best to try presenting without them at first, then decide if they are needed. Prices have increased with the extra demand for online presentations, especially during the COVID-19 pandemic, and some items are likely to remain difficult to get hold of for some time. In any case, the most popular brands are not essential for an adequate setup, and the most pragmatic approach is to try out the equipment you currently have, supplementing it only if really necessary. An extra lighting source is needed, but the precise type to use is of secondary importance. The equipment and setup should make you feel more confident that you can present well, and this confidence will then translate into a superior presentation [1].

4.3   Presentation Software Applications

The fact that PowerPoint is so ubiquitous for presentations has meant, paradoxically, that many presentations seem dull repeats of other presentations. A set of slides that consists simply of bullet-point lists is not likely to garner significant attention. Thus, whilst PowerPoint definitely has a place in presentations, it need not be the only software for presenters to consider using. Other applications are also effective for conveying a message in a presentation.

PowerPoint is similar to Keynote and Google Slides, all of which can be used to put together a slide deck. All these tools are more impressive if there is variation from the list format, by use of images or animations, and by keeping any text-based elements as short and concise as possible.

The following sections detail tools which are all suitable for presentations and may help to make the presentation even more enjoyable and engaging.

4.3.1   Visme

Visme is an application that works in the cloud. Its emphasis is on facilitating presentations with a major visual element to get the audience's attention and let you put your message across. The interface utilises a drag-and-drop method, which most people find highly intuitive. The professional version of the service offers tools to make the branding consistent across presentations and lets images be stored where the whole company staff have access. Once set up, employees can create a presentation which has the officially approved colour scheme and logos. Thus, different presentations will be clearly related to the same brand. Furthermore, Visme comes with an integral capacity to perform analysis of who watched the presentation and how much of it they actually saw.

Visme has a series of different pricing options and offers the possibility of a live demonstration of the application's capabilities, at no cost to potential clients.

4.3.2   Haiku Deck

Haiku Deck is marketed as a presentation aid that is as simple to use as possible. It can be used to produce slides which are elegant and graced with images of the highest quality. The aim of the simple approach is to emphasise engagement with the audience over delivering a large volume of information. The particular strength of Haiku Deck lies in its very extensive image library and the multiple fonts available. Presentations which play well on any device and are highly effective can be created easily.

The pricing options for this web-based solution include various monthly plans [3].

4.3.3   Pitcherific

Pitcherific is more than simply a tool for assembling a set of presentation slides. It also helps with designing what you want to say and giving you practice saying it. There are multiple templates, and the application guides users step-by-step through the preparation of a suitable presentation. The focus is on what you are going to say, rather than writing content for the accompanying slides. The template for a so-called elevator pitch breaks down the process into the creation of the hook, outlining the problem you are offering to solve, the solution you propose and the way to close your pitch. There is a rich variety of different templates to cover multiple different presentation types. As well as guiding you through what to say, Pitcherific also provides guidance on how long a section should last and the number of words to include, as well as letting you time yourself. In this way, the presentation should always be the optimal length.

The pricing for Pitcherific is determined by the type of company you work for and what the precise needs of the company are. Therefore, pricing information is best obtained directly from a Pitcherific sales agent. There are, however, demonstrations of the platform available at no cost [3].

4.3.4 Canva

Canva is a web-based service that helps with producing a variety of materials that may be needed in a business context, such as CVs, newsletters, press releases, brochures, infographics and business cards. In addition to these materials, there are several hundred different templates to create a slide deck for a presentation. Canva has over a million images that can be used in the creation of materials, or users can upload their own images. Within each template, it is easy to change text appearance, filter images and design the visual layout using a drag and drop interface. The business logo can be uploaded to be used on branded materials.

Canva offers a no-cost version of the application, which is suitable for newly beginning businesses or ones which have few employees. As the business grows, the paid version (Canva for Work) may be more suitable, as it includes ways to work with teams. There are monthly pricing options and the professional version is free for the first 30 days of use [3].

4.3.5 SlideCamp

SlideCamp is a solution for businesses which need to maintain a consistent look-and-feel for presentations produced by different departments. It offers multiple templates which can be customised for the appropriate colour scheme and logo to display. Data, including graphical representations, can be uploaded. The slides can also be assigned to different sections of a presentation. Once the details of branding have been confirmed on SlideCamp, other employees will be able to create slides which have a very professional appearance. This tool is mostly suitable for business of at least medium size, with a pricing structure which reflects that fact. It may be an expensive option if the company buying the service is small.

The exact cost depends on the number of licensed users required, although the range is between 50 and 500 USD at the time of writing. A demonstration version of the software can also be tried out before committing to a purchase [3].

4.3.6 Microsoft Events

PowerPoint has lost something of the freshness it once had as presentation software, but Microsoft has recently brought out a range of different functionalities in its

Microsoft 365 package. One of these new functionalities is the ability to produce a live session, or to host an on-demand presentation. The live events can be viewed when they are being presented, perhaps by colleagues in remote locations, or afterwards to catch up on what information was shared. The packages offer high definition video and use artificial intelligence techniques to generate a speaker timeline, a transcript and time stamps. Closed captioning is also available.

Since access to these functionalities is already included in a subscription for Office 365, there is no need to pay extra for these features [3].

4.3.7   Powtoon

Powtoon is a service allowing its users to create animations and videos to use as presentations. The format is suitable for creating promotional or explainer videos. This kind of video presentation is a key way to increase brand awareness about your product and to reach new customers or clients. Powtoon permits this in an affordable way. With this platform, users can edit a presentation or video easily. Voiceovers can also be added to video. The results look very professional and are impressive for clients.

In terms of pricing, the service does have a cost-free version, but greater functionality is available with a paid subscription, which ranges in price from around 20 to 60 USD each month [3].

4.3.8   VideoScribe

The VideoScribe platform is targeted mainly at small businesses which need to produce explainer or marketing videos in an easy way. It takes the form of a virtual whiteboard with a hand that appears to draw or write the video, as ordinary human presenters might draw on a whiteboard to explain some concept. The interface is straightforward and permits text, images and drawings to be included in the presentation. Users can also draw their own objects using VideoScribe.

The pricing options include an individual user licence (1 month or repeating monthly subscription), team licence or a lifetime licence [3]. The latest details on pricing can be seen on the VideoScribe website [4].

4.3.9   Prezi

Prezi is a web-based application that allows the creation of slides from templates. However, what gives the resulting presentations greater impact is the way the slides move from one to another. The software creates a map of the entire presentation and lets you choose how you wish to navigate through it. As the presentation moves forward, the audience can also see the order in which you are presenting the material. Thus the audience gets a better overview of how the subjects in a presentation are related to each other. Different slides can be assigned to particular sections, and an overview setup to show the audience the whole presentation at one glance. In this way, the presentation remains coherent and the audience remain interested. Note that the path you set up through the presentation may be deviated from as required. It is not fixed.

The latest pricing options can be seen on the Prezi website [5].

4.4   In Which Ways Do Online Presentations Differ from F2F?

Although it might be argued that the same features that make an F2F presentation successful also exist in online presentations, there are significant differences between the two formats. They call for different techniques to maximise audience engagement. There are two aspects, in particular, which differ between online and F2F presentations [6], namely:

4.4.1   Audiences Watching Online Presentations Experience Greater Distractions than Is Usual in an F2F Setting

If an audience member is viewing a presentation online, the environment differs considerably from the case where the audience all sit together in the same room for an F2F presentation. The absence of distractions in an F2F environment means the presenter does not need to work so hard to keep the audience focused on the presentation. The audience in an F2F setting naturally pays attention to the speaker's body language. The online presentation is a rather different setting overall.

For a start, usually the audience will be watching with their own sound (and possibly video, too) switched off. Thus the presenter misses those usual cues that indicate whether the audience are engaged and following what is being said. In this situation, the audience members may easily be only half-listening to the presenter whilst trying to catch up on e-mails, making calls, looking at LinkedIn or Facebook or just idly clock watching, waiting for the work to finish [6]. The presenter cannot tell what the real audience situation is.

4.4.2   Online Presenting Can Be Easily Scaled Up, Unlike F2F

Presentations delivered online can be easily streamed to very large audiences, up to hundreds of individuals. There are many videoconferencing solutions that allow a large audience to be involved. One such solution is offered by Lifesize [7]. For individuals to attend an online presentation, they may need nothing more than an internet connection and the link to the meeting. Thus attendance becomes much easier to arrange than for F2F meetings, where travel is typically required, time away from the office may need to be authorised and a venue arranged. Even with the best laid plans, the presenter can still not be sure of who will actually attend until the day of the event itself.

However, whilst attending an online presentation does offer various advantages in terms of convenience, it would be a mistake to assume that every aspect will be more straightforward for both the presenter and the audience. Unfortunately, online presentations do regularly fail to live up to expectations through having poor quality sound or video, or through the presenter's unfamiliarity with using the technology involved. To establish rapport and engage an audience online, furthermore, requires even more effort on the part of the presenter than in an F2F meeting.

The next sections outline specific advice for how to establish rapport and engage your audience when presenting virtually [6].

4.5   Advice for How to Present Online

All presentations, whether online or F2F, call for excellence in content, speaker preparation and delivery. Online presentations, however, stand or fall by whether the presenter is able to eliminate unnecessary distractions or not. The following four sections give advice on how online presenters can reduce distractions to an absolute minimum [6].

4.5.1   Be Brief

Audiences attending an online presentation are especially prone to being distracted, whether by receiving e-mail, WhatsApp notifications or by social media updates. Given this reality, the presentation needs to be kept as brief, succinct and readily understandable as possible. Should the presentation be a long one, such as when chairing a webinar, it is vital to stick to the key topic and not get lost in the details.

On average, an audience member can concentrate properly on what a speaker is saying for between 5 and 10 min. However skilled a presenter is, to keep the audience properly focused on a presentation for a period exceeding 20 min is extremely difficult. To stop the audience getting tired and to keep them focused, the presentation needs to hit hard, with a maximum of five essential messages, and be capable of being condensed into a succinct take home message.

A practical way to make sure your presentation is of this kind is to set an objective for the presentation first, before you start adding content. Thus, a presentation that offers advice on increasing productivity when working remotely may have the objective of getting the audience to try out the advice and report back. This will then determine what content should be included, i.e. whatever is necessary to equip them with the new skills [6].

4.5.2   Shut Down Unused Windows First

It is important that when you initiate screen sharing, the presentation should appear without delay and that no other windows are inadvertently shared. If there are too many windows open, it is easy to share the wrong window, which not only looks unprepared, it also runs the risk of sharing private information, such as e-mails. When the presentation opens smoothly as expected, the audience's attention will be captured straightaway and the first impression about the presenter will be positive.

Another important misstep to avoid is failing to separate out the exact slides you want to present from a larger selection. Often a presentation may need to be delivered to a number of separate audiences, with some overlap of information. Therefore, some people prefer to use a large master presentation slide set, from which they can select the sections of most relevance to the particular audience. The danger in this approach is that a presenter may show irrelevant slides, which will cause the audience to rapidly lose interest. Thus, attention should be paid to separating out the most appropriate slides and presenting them in a smooth progression to avoid breaks in the audience's focus [6].

4.5.3   Get the Audience to Co-operate in Reducing Distractions

It is common for employees of companies which use remote working extensively to mute themselves when they are attending a conference. There are few things as embarrassing or distracting as background noise during a presentation. When the time comes for interaction, the presenter can ask the audience to unmute themselves. In some cases, the host can actually mute other participants, which may offer a greater degree of control. Keeping participants on mute until they are in line to speak helps to maintain everyone's focus.

Another rule in some companies is to get the audience to turn any mobile devices to silent and avoid answering messages during a presentation. In this way, even though the audience are remotely located, they are more like participants in an F2F meeting, who should normally avoid answering the telephone during a presentation [6].

4.5.4   Run a Check on the Equipment Before the Event Starts

Most people who have watched a few online presentations have seen the awkward situation where a presenter is speaking, but no sound comes because he/she forgot to unmute the microphone first, or where the content fails to appear to the audience due to incorrect screen sharing. Whilst these mishaps are common, with some basic precautions taken, they need not occur.

The first precaution is to do a check on the working condition of the microphone, screen sharing and video camera a quarter of an hour before the time the presentation is due to start. At this point, any technical hitches can be identified and, all being well, corrected. At the same time, it is worth checking the illumination levels in the room where you will present, to see if it looks appropriate on the webcast.

Even if everything is working as expected, this is still time well-spent, since it gives you confidence that there are unlikely to be any technical problems during the presentation [6].

4.6 Presentation Technique with Lifesize

One particularly effective application that can be used for videoconferencing, offering a high level of security and reliability, as well as offering a great user experience, is Lifesize. This solution works well on many different systems and devices. The following advice is specially tailored for presenters using Lifesize [6].

4.6.1 Prepare a Suitable Presentation

All presentations need to consist of engaging text and visual elements. For commercial presentations, useful material may already exist which can be copied from the company website, official blog or social media offerings.

When the content of the presentation is well-written, the presentation will be more convincing. Stress how taking action will benefit the audience, offer answers to common objections and challenge your audience to take action. This way the audience will get engaged in the presentation.

If a presentation is especially important, it may be wise to involve a professional copywriter, who can draft slides that have the maximum positive impact on an audience and spur them into action. The tools which are now available to make creating a presentation a more interactive process, such as Visme, mean that now it is much more straightforward to prepare a presentation with a unique appeal and one which engages the audience deeply. Visme also offers tips and advice regularly on the ideal ways to create a presentation that does not suffer from information overload [6].

4.6.2 Choose the "Present" Option

Once the presentation has been assembled and the meeting time arrives, choose the option within the application to present, which brings you into the Lifesize meeting. Check that everyone you are expecting has arrived, then share your screen to begin. Lifesize asks you which window you wish to share.

4.6.3   Sharing May Involve Just the Slides or the Whole Screen

Having chosen which windows you want to share, click to confirm the selection, then you will be ready to begin. It is important to make sure any other presenters have finished screen sharing before you attempt to do so [6].

4.7   Actions to Take Following a Presentation

Once the presentation is complete, you can feel relieved, but this point is also an opportunity to reflect on your own performance as a presenter and to think about any improvements you may make next time. It is also good practice to request some feedback from colleagues who were present. This is a way to see whether the objective of the presentation was met. Additionally, there are several further steps which can help ensure that a well-delivered presentation converts into real return for the business [6].

4.7.1   Distribute a Link Where People Can See the Recorded Session

In some cases, the audience may want to watch the presentation a second time to ensure they understand all the information you gave them. Lifesize is well set up to permit recording. After the recording is finished, you can easily share it by forwarding a link to interested parties. The video recording can also be edited with appropriate software to use in future sessions, such as webinars, teleconferences or other kinds of meetings.

4.7.2   Where Needed, Book in Follow-Up Sessions

You can define a suitable time for a follow-up meeting, but there is no advantage in waiting to book it in with the client. It is an indication of a successful online meeting that it ends with a commitment to a further follow-up meeting. By following up prospective or actual clients, you keep your offer fresh in their minds and can make sure there are no delays or missteps in completion of any joint projects [6].

4.8   FAQs Regarding Online Presentations

4.8.1   How Are Online Presentations Assembled?

There are applications to allow a set of slides and appropriate visuals to be gathered into a presentation. An example is PowerPoint or Impress. There should also be a meeting software application, such as Zoom or Lifesize. This software allows presenters to share their screen. The final element is simply deciding what you want to say as you show the slides.

4.8.2   What Is the Way to Engage Audiences When Presenting Online?

Maximum audience engagement occurs with presentations that move smoothly forward accompanied by appropriate comments for each slide. Presenters should speak enthusiastically and persuasively whilst also providing opportunities for the audience to ask questions so that they can remain interested in what you have to say.

4.8.3   What Kinds of Problems Should Online Presenters Be Prepared to Face?

The main unpredictable element in online presenting is technical failure. The signal may be delayed, the video or sound may be "choppy" and the connection may get dropped unexpectedly. When there is a dedicated videoconferencing application available, the principal issue will probably be keeping the audience focused on the presentation despite the many potential distractions that occur in this situation [6].

References

1. Brownlee D. Presenting virtually? Here are the 4 home office items you need. https://www.forbes.com/sites/danabrownlee/2020/05/13/presenting-virtually-here-are-the-4-home-office-items-you-need/?sh=52a296e324cd. Accessed 3 Oct 2021.
2. How to get rid of pesky ring light reflection in your glasses! https://www.juliamaephotography.com/blog/how-to-get-rid-of-pesky-ring-light-reflection-in-your-glasses/. Accessed 24 Oct 2021.
3. D'Angelo M. Beyond PowerPoint: presentation tools for small businesses. 2018. https://www.businessnewsdaily.com/6525-business-presentation-tools.html. Accessed 3 Oct 2021.
4. Whiteboard animation pricing. https://www.videoscribe.co/en/pricing/. Accessed 26 Oct 2021.
5. Prezi pricing. https://prezi.com/0ciftoyy5g-n/prezi-pricing/. Accessed 26 Oct 2021.
6. Yarbrough J. How to give a virtual presentation: tips, challenges, and more. 2020. https://www.lifesize.com/en/blog/virtual-presentation-tips/. Accessed 3 Oct 2021.
7. Lifesize. https://www.lifesize.com/en/. Accessed 26 Oct 2021.

Preparation and Planning

5

5.1 Make Sure You Know the Brief

It is vital, just as in any project or task, to understand at the beginning what you are expected to do prior to beginning the preparation phase. Look carefully at the requirements for the presentation, with the following questions in mind [1]:

- Will the audience consist of one person or several?
- What are the constraints on timing?
- Is it permissible to show video during the presentation? If it is, what length is acceptable? For the majority of presentations, videos will need to be fairly short and with clear relevance to the topic being presented.
- What is the main subject to cover? Is there some discretion allowed regarding the title?
- Should the presentation be accompanied by visual aids, such as slides or a poster?
- Why are you presenting the particular topic? Is it designed to update your peers or educate colleagues? Is the aim to present the results of marketing research or a scientific trial? Is the aim to present a persuasive case? Or is the presentation a synopsis of a literary work?

5.2 Making a Plan

Preparation is an indispensable step in delivering a high-quality presentation. Typically, the following processes are required to maximise the chances of success [1]:

- Brainstorming for ideas and deciding on a broad outline. What does the topic actually cover? What information is already at your fingertips? What do you aim for the audience to learn from the presentation?

© The Author(s), under exclusive license to Springer Nature
Switzerland AG 2023
C. C. Cingi et al., *Improving Online Presentations*,
https://doi.org/10.1007/978-3-031-28328-4_5

- Researching facts and statistics which bolster your argument. Reading around the topic so as to be familiar with the subject area.
- Writing down the key points.
- Preparing a draft version.
- Consideration of how you intend to use visual aids, such as the use of PowerPoint or other presentation software. Deciding on any interactivity you wish to include.
- Practising the presentation several times, removing any sections or extra words that slow you down. Remembering to check you can conform to the time limit.

5.3   Stages of Preparation for Presentations

As described above, there are several processes involved in preparing to present. These processes or stages can be categorised under the following seven headings [2]:

1. Choice of subject
2. Defining the aims
3. Information gathering
4. Producing the overall plan or preparing a script to follow
5. Selection of visual elements
6. Picking an appropriate title
7. Practising delivery

Since there are so many different formats for delivering a presentation, not every presentation will involve all seven activities. For example, a speech does not call for selection of visual elements. An elevator pitch may also need to be assembled quickly if an opportunity to pitch a product or idea crops up. Nonetheless, for any presentation, the more time you can devote to preparation, the higher the likelihood that the presentation will be successful [2].

5.3.1   First Stage: Choice of Subject

The choice of subject is the single most essential stage when preparing a presentation. If the topic is something that the presenter has little interest in or enthusiasm for, it is unlikely that the presentation will hit the right note. It is important to be enthusiastic about the subject you choose, since interest is a powerful motivator to undertake the stages of preparation in a sufficiently thorough way. Lack of interest in a topic is virtually impossible to hide when you come to deliver the presentation. If the choice is free, there are multiple ways to look at a topic and angles from which to present. It is important, however, not to keep delivering the same presentation for year after year. The topic must also be suitable for the expected audience. It is advisable to be even-handed when presenting, rather than fiercely partisan, which may alienate the audience. Ensure that the topic or angle matches your knowledge and ability in a subject. Thus, whenever possible, choose subjects that are already somewhat familiar to you. Familiarity with the basic facts means you can concentrate instead on the angle from which you intend to approach the topic. A familiar subject is also easier to discuss when questions are asked by the audience members. That said, experienced presenters should stretch themselves, whether by extending their existing knowledge or by coming at the topic from a novel direction. Experiment with different formats. It is often said that the best way to learn a subject is to teach it, so preparing a presentation is a chance for self-development. It is not always necessary to pick an edgy topic to generate interest. The approach you take can make even a familiar topic fresh and thought-provoking. For example, you might supply surprising facts about a familiar topic.

Topics should be neither too restricted nor too general. A very general topic may lack focus and a presentation may seem to just skim over the surface, leaving the audience unsatisfied. A very restricted topic, however, may seem too slight to interest the audience and there may be insufficient material to fill the time. A biochemist might find that a presentation on "laboratory methods" would be too broad to do justice to, whilst "Southern blotting" may be too narrow. A compromise might be something like "electrophoresis techniques in the laboratory". Or "French cuisine" may be too massive to discuss in a single session, whilst "Crème brûlée" is too limited. How about "Top ten French desserts"? The availability of suitable visuals may also limit the choice.

It is also important to tailor the presentation to the audience. A presentation about 1980s personal computers might focus more on nostalgia if it were to be delivered to a general audience but would call for more technical detail if presented to the Computer Society. The level of detail should not be such as to "blind the audience with science".

The number of potential audience members is also a key factor to consider, if there is to be a practical demonstration. The entire audience needs to be able to see what is happening. Plan in such a way that this is possible.

Finally, if brainstorming does not lead to a topic, you can always ask friends, peers or colleagues for suggestions. Nonetheless, wherever possible, presenters should choose their own topic and title. There are suggestions for suitable titles to use for a variety of topics in other chapters of this book.

5.3.2 Second Stage: Defining the Aims

Having reached a decision on the topic to present, the next thing to consider is the best format for the presentation. Presenters may work singly or in groups. The choice of one or several presenters depends on the topic you have chosen. Consider the content you plan to include and think about the optimal way to put the message across. The goal or objective of the presentation should guide your thoughts about how to deliver. What response are you aiming for from your audience? Is the goal to instruct the audience in a technical procedure? If so, how detailed will the instruction be? If a demonstration is involved, will there be a product at the end to see?

Going back to our hypothetical French desserts presentation, will there be chance to see a completed dessert, maybe even taste it?

Many presentations are intended to provide information to the audience or to educate them in some way. Consider whether visual aids can help ("a picture is worth a thousand words"). To what extent will time limits restrict the information you can provide? Are there practical limitations to a demonstration that mean a slideshow is more appropriate? Conversely, the speech format may be ideal if the aim is not about educating the listeners or informing them, but to spur them into action. Politicians do not usually use slides but concentrate more on persuasive rhetoric.

5.3.3 Third Stage: Information Gathering

At the information gathering stage, the aim is to ensure the presenter knows the subject as well as possible first. A time-frame of at least 1 month is ideal for this stage. Being well-versed in the subject will translate into a more confident performance during Q and As. This stage of preparation is vital; otherwise, the presenter will fail to be truly impressive. Audiences can readily realise when a presenter is fumbling for an answer or avoiding a question. The information gathering stage may involve consulting any or all of the following: textbooks, journals, popular magazines, industry reports, websites, documentary programmes, expert opinions and your own personal experience, amongst other resources.

Remember to keep track of where you sourced any material you intend to use in the presentation. References are important, so that the reliability of the source can be verified by interested parties. Information should be up-to-date and accurate. Furthermore, it is important to distinguish between factual information and opinions. The former can be shown to be objectively true, whereas an opinion reflects someone's judgement. If you quote an opinion, try to get other opinions to compare it with.

Keeping track of references can be done in various ways. The traditional way is to keep a card index with the quote/fact and the source clearly indicated. However, there are now a number of software applications specially designed to help with keeping track of references. Even just keeping the references in a single word processed file may be sufficient if there are not too many entries. References can then be included in the presentation, as footnotes or endnotes. Referencing a presentation is essential to avoid plagiarism and to establish how reliable your information is.

5.3.4 Fourth Step: Prepare an Outline or Script

Preparing the words you plan to use whilst delivering your presentation can be done in numerous ways. For some presenters, a few notes forming an outline are sufficient, whilst others want to actually script the words they intend to use at the beginning and end of the presentation. In a few cases, a presenter may prefer to write a script for the entire presentation. It is best to practise delivering the presentation in various ways, then decide which works best. However you decide to proceed, the initial action to take is to compose an outline with the main points included and to decide on the order in which you will present each point. Prepare the headings you need to order the material and arrange what to place under each heading. Decide what visual elements are to be included. The following are sample outlines for a demonstration presentation and an illustrated talk. They can be used as models [2]:

1. Introduction
    (a) Icebreaker
    (b) Self-introduction
    (c) Preview of the actual demonstration
2. Body of presentation
    (a) First step. Includes reason for performing step plus method to use
    (b) Second step. Ditto
    (c) Third step. Ditto
    (d) Show the result/finished product
3. Conclusion
    (a) Repeat steps in summarised form
    (b) End with an unexpected twist
    (c) Give references [2]

5.3.4.1 Illustrated Speech or Talk

1. Introduction
    (a) Icebreaker
    (b) Self-introduction
    (c) Overview of topics to be covered
2. Body of presentation
    (a) Key message #1
            Related visuals (images, diagrams, etc.)
            Supporting evidence
    (b) Key message #2
            Related visuals (images, diagrams, etc.)
            Supporting evidence
    (c) Key message #3
            Related visuals (images, diagrams, etc.)
            Supporting evidence
3. Concluding section
    (a) Summarise the messages
    (b) Attention-grabbing final remarks
    (c) Quote resources used [2]

With the outline now filled out, you can start to prepare the entire presentation. However, the best way to do so is not, as many people do, to start at the introduction. It is actually more straightforward to complete the body section of the presentation first. That way, you will be much clearer on exactly what you intend to cover. The next stage is to sketch out your concluding remarks, and only at the end do you turn to writing the introduction. This method is the most practical for ensuring the whole presentation fits together properly. Experiment with different ways to explain the key points and write down any particular phrases that seem especially apposite. This stage involves several iterations before the ideal wording is established. For presenters who want to script the presentation in its entirety, the script should be longer than you initially anticipate. Omitting a few paragraphs is always easier than trying to extemporise a script on the day. Once the script is written, leave it for a day or two before re-reading it and making any amendments. The script can then be sorted out into sections written on cue cards. The best type of language is always vivid and lively but should not be too complex. Where technical terms are needed, ensure you define your terms. Slang expressions are best avoided altogether. Try to speak in a descriptive way, so that the audience can more easily imagine what you are describing. It is generally easier for an audience to grasp "just over a half" than "0.509". Structure your discourse with pointer and transition terms or conjugations: "next", "before that", "now". These words establish a clearer structure for the audience. Be careful, however, not to keep repeating the same word, "next...next...next", as this becomes tedious.

Whilst practising the presentation, it is important to consider more than just the script. Just as an actor needs to remember the "blocking" (the movements which accompany the words), so presenters need to think about any gestures to employ, how to use the visual aids and any actions that accompany a demonstration. For a speech, in particular, it is important to rehearse the accompanying gestures, tone of voice and the accompanying movements you will make. Use the cue cards at first, but as you become more familiar with the presentation, keep simplifying the cue cards. Decide what are the most vital points to emphasise and highlight them on the cards so that you easily see those points when you glance at the cards. All being well, after some practice the cue cards will no longer be needed. Remember, nonetheless, to write a number on the top of each card, so that you can find the appropriate card if your memory goes blank in the presentation and you need a reminder [2].

5.3.5 Fifth Stage: Choose What Visuals You Want to Include

Visual elements of many different kinds can complement the words used in a presentation. Videos, infographics, slides, animations and others all add interest. Samples of products or other real objects may be shown. For a demonstration, some type of illustration is essential. The speech format generally does not allow for visual aids. In most presentations, however, having a visual element improves the presentation, increasing interest and engagement by the listeners. Furthermore, most people benefit greatly from visual understanding. "Seeing", as the saying goes, "is believing". Indeed, carefully selected visual aids are often what differentiates a high quality from an indifferent presentation. But such aids must be relevant and suitable to illustrate the point you are making, not merely decorative.

When a visual aid is to be used, it needs to be readily visible. The visual aid should not distract from the main thrust of the presentation. Avoid demonstrating objects that are difficult to handle or which are so minute that the audience strains to see them. The visual elements should fit seamlessly into the presentation, assisting delivery of your key message or messages [2].

5.3.6   Sixth Stage: Choice of Title

Once the plan for the content and delivery of the presentation has been finalised, you will need to come up with a title that can grab the potential audience's attention. A powerful title conveys the idea that the presentation will be worth listening to and stimulates the audience's curiosity. An effective title makes clear what the topic will be, but without stealing the presenter's thunder. Thus, it is well worth the effort spent considering different options. Creativity and originality are called for. Generally speaking, a title that works well will possess at least one of the following characteristics [2]:

- It is brief and highly relevant
- It describes the topic
- It is thought-provoking
- It generates an image in the mind of the listener
- It conveys a sense of enjoyment

The following are examples of how to convert a dull-sounding title into a better one:

- Safety Precautions When Horse Riding vs Staying Safe in the Saddle
- Recipes Involving Apples vs Appletastic Delight
- How to Groom a Scruffy Dog vs Make Your Best Friend a Handsome Hound
- Rewilding National Parks vs Bringing Back the Great Wilderness
- Elementary Care of Reptiles vs Snakes and Adders for Beginners

5.3.7   Seventh Stage: Practising

All your effort expended in preparing a knock-out presentation will be wasted unless you remember to practise the presentation thoroughly before you deliver it for real. Presenters who spend time practising always feel better prepared and sure of their ability to present.

However, there is a difference between practising a presentation and learning it completely by heart. The aim of practising is to make the material familiar enough that you can present it in a natural-sounding way. You may wish to use cue cards at first but aim to be able to present without them following practice. Furthermore, whilst practising, speak out loud, so you can really hear how it sounds. Practise saying everything you will in the real presentation, so that you are not left struggling for words mid-sentence. By going through the whole presentation each time you practise, you can ensure each section follows on naturally from the preceding one and gain an idea of exactly how long delivery of the presentation takes. Think about what the audience may ask and be prepared to give good answers. Where visual aids are involved, ensure you know how to present them. The script needs to be synchronised with the appropriate visuals. If you have items to show, lay them out in the order in which they will be used whilst presenting. Check how to use any applications, such as a virtual whiteboard. By becoming familiar with the actual equipment you will use, your presentation will not be derailed by you struggling to get some piece of equipment to work the way you want. Wherever and whenever possible, practise in front of an audience of trusted family or friends, who can advise on how the presentation appears and may be suggest areas for improvement. Additionally, by practising whilst videoing yourself, or in front of a mirror, you can observe whether your body language and gestures match the message. If it is possible, practise delivery in different places, to get used to unfamiliar environments. Finally, aim to do the last practice one or 2 h before actual delivery, so that the order and way to present are firmly rooted in your memory [2].

References

1. Giving presentations. https://columbiacollege-ca.libguides.com/presentations/planning. Accessed 4 Oct 2021.
2. Steps in planning a presentation. Oregon State University. https://extension.oregonstate.edu/sites/default/files/documents/10551/stepsinplanningapresentation.pdf. Accessed 4 Oct 2021.

6.1 Introduction

High-quality presentations follow a logical, coherent order, with an identifiable beginning, body and conclusion.

6.1.1 The Beginning (Introduction)

The first part of the presentation is of vital importance, since this is the chance to get the listeners focused on yourself and the topic and to establish the approach you will adopt.

- Include an "attention grabber", such as posing a challenge, displaying an image that makes the audience curious, telling a tale or relating an example from real life, revealing a surprising statistic, delivering a pithy quote or perhaps playing a brief video.
- Introduce yourself and clearly state the subject(s) to be covered.
- Provide an overview of what you will discuss [1].

6.1.2 Body of the Presentation

- Introduce the information in a logically coherent way.
- Transitions from one topic to another should be clearly signalled.
- Remember to back up points with specific examples [1].

C. C. Cingi et al., *Improving Online Presentations*,
https://doi.org/10.1007/978-3-031-28328-4_6

6.1.3   Conclusion

- Provide a summary of what has been presented
- New topics or information should not be introduced in the conclusion, but it is acceptable to pose questions that you want the audience to consider following your presentation.
- Use language to signal that you are drawing the presentation to a close, but avoid an abrupt statement like, "the end".
- Do not be tempted to apologise for using up your audience's time.
- Remember to thank your listeners for their attention and prompt them to ask any questions [1].

6.2   Words and Phrases to Signal Transitions

Words and phrases that signal a transition are valuable in making the structure of a presentation clearly visible and helping to guide the listeners through the material. The following sections provide useful phrases that can be used to signal a transition [1].

6.2.1   In the Introduction

- *Today I will be looking at …*
- *The presentation will cover the following topics …*

6.2.2   Explaining the Outline or Overview of the Presentation

- *I would like to begin with … followed by …*
- *The talk consists of four (five, six etc.) sections. We start with … after which … leading to … and finally we will discuss …*
- *There are three key themes I wish to talk about, namely A, B and C*
- *Let's start by discussing … then we can move onto …* [1]

6.2.3   Highlighting the Key Message(s) of the Presentation

- *One of the key problems concerns …*
- *A significant factor to consider is …*
- *The principal issue relates to …* [1]

6.2.4   Paraphrasing for Emphasis

- *To put it another way …*
- *Or we can say it like this: the main issue is …*

6.2.5   Transitioning Between Topics

- *Let us now think about …*
- *We now need to turn to …*
- *The next issue we can think about is …*

6.2.6   How to Introduce a Specific Example

- *We can illustrate this by looking at …*
- *Consider what happened last year …*
- *A good illustration of this is provided by ….*
- *Let me give you a specific example …* [1]

6.2.7   Talking About Visual Elements or Illustrations

- *This is a diagram showing …*
- *From the picture, we can observe how …* [1]

6.2.8   Introducing and Explaining Video Clips

- *I would like to show you a brief clip showing …*
- *As you saw in the clip, a key point to note is …*
- *Just as we saw in the video …* [1]

6.2.9   Concluding Phrases

- *So, in summary …*
- *We can thus conclude …*
- *The conclusion is …*
- *Summarising, we can say …*
- *Putting it all together …*
- *Finally …* [1]

6.2.10 Inviting and Responding to Questions

- *We now have some space for questions. Who wants to start?*
- *Thank you. Your question raises an interesting point …*
- *Great question. What the data indicate is that …*
- *Thanks for that question. I think it goes beyond my presentation today, but maybe we can keep if for another time?*
- *Unfortunately, I don't have the information to answer that at present, but it is an issue to think about in the future, certainly.*

6.3   Assembling the Presentation

6.3.1   Gathering High-Quality Information to Present

6.3.1.1   Consider Your Objective in the Presentation

When you come to put a presentation together, it is essential to consider your objective in presenting first. See the presentation as an opportunity to put across a specific message (or messages) and order the material in the most efficient way to achieve this goal [2, 3].

- Put down in writing the most essential points you wish to get across and decide if a central theme emerges. What is the unique "take home message" that you are aiming for?
- Be careful not to "blind your audience with science". Facts should only be provided in context and organised so that they convey meaning. Consider how data or other facts support or reinforce your message.

6.3.1.2   Be Aware What Background Your Listeners Have and Tailor the Presentation to Suit Them

Unless your presentation covers a topic you already expect your audience to be familiar with, you will need to provide the basic material needed to grasp the issues and comprehend your message. Think carefully about what the likely expectations of the listeners will be. Consider how this intersects with your objective, such as [4]:

- If you are attempting to do a sales pitch, inform the audience about a new concept or change the way they think, what information do they need to possess to do so?
- Consider the personalities involved. Does the audience consist of individuals who are likely to be difficult to win over, or are they already on your side and looking forward to hearing what comes next?

6.3.1.3 The Length of the Presentation Governs What You Can Present

Choose carefully the data, information or facts that allow you best to convey your message, according to the time you have available. In a 10-min presentation, the maximum number of key points you can cover is three. Note how each point is connected to the other points and prepare a logical structure of presentation. Be aware that sometimes you will need to discuss points that are not naturally connected to each other [5]. Be careful not to include too much information. For instance, if you wish to persuade a firm to take part in a recycling initiative, it would probably be relevant to touch on the effects of corporate waste on global warming, as well as the economic impact recycling can make on the bottom line. However, the melting of polar ice, whilst certainly a consequence of global warming, would be too far removed from the central objective to justify inclusion in the presentation [2].

6.3.1.4 Identify the Information or Data that Offer the Best Support to Your Argument

Sift carefully through the results of your research to identify those facts and figures that bolster the message. Material you include should be thought-provoking and likely to motivate the audience to act. Information that you include in your presentation fulfils one or more of the following purposes [5]:

- It helps to clarify the message by providing explanation and illustration. A brief thumbnail sketch might, for example, summarise how greenhouse gases produce global warming.
- It helps to justify your viewpoint, by linking in findings from experimental studies, polls or other research. The recycling presentation discussed above would, for instance, benefit from a slide showing how well the theory of global warming is supported by the accumulating evidence and how widely scientists agree with its conclusions.
- It adds visual interest by including images, videos, charts or diagrams. As an example, a colourful infographic illustrating how waste can be recycled would add interest to the corporate recycling programme presentation.

6.3.2 Establishing the Route You Intend to Follow

6.3.2.1 Begin Strongly with a Well-Crafted Introduction

Following on from selection of the most appropriate material, work can begin on preparing an outline/route map through the material. The first part of any successful presentation is a powerful introduction, which immediately engages the audience in the topic [6].

- Remember to introduce yourself, stating your name, any affiliations and mentioning your credentials, for example, "I'm Archie Hope, Head of Marketing at Ulusoy Aesthetics. I have been managing online communication and consulting with surgery candidates for the last two years. Today I would like to discuss …"
- Focus the attention of your listeners by getting them to think about an interesting problem or puzzling fact: "Do you know why so many people are coming to our country for aesthetic procedures such as hair transplants, rhinoplasty, and others?"
- There is no need to compose the presentation in the order in which you will finally present it. Indeed, it may be better to compose the introduction at a later date, as explained in Chap. 5.

6.3.2.2 The Body of the Presentation Is the Place to Lay Out the Results of Your Research

The body portion typically accounts for between two-thirds and three-quarters of the presentation, and this is where the key points are to be found. The body should be a series of signposts on the way to a conclusion. Accordingly, the material needs to be laid out in a logically and coherently structured fashion. One way is to present an issue, outline what further problems the issue may cause and then move towards a potential solution [6]. For the aesthetic surgery promotion presentation, this may take the following form:

- Start by setting the problems of the ageing face. Show that this is an issue that affects millions of people.
- Outline what happens when this problem is not addressed on time. Give evidence that supports the idea that the procedures and costs will increase if not performed immediately. Then introduce the idea that it is possible to prevent these unwanted consequences by taking a specific action, i.e. joining the scheme you are proposing, such as using creams, injections or surgery [2]. Note that the audience's reaching the decision to join the scheme was the objective in you presenting.

6.3.2.3 Linking Statements Are Helpful in Clarifying the Argument

Linking statements are phrases that show how one idea is joined to another and facilitate the presenter moving from point to point. They help the audience to perceive the structure of the presentation, making it easier to understand [5].

- Some examples of linking statements are as follows: "That brings us to the next issue …", "We now turn to what happens when …" and "Let's move on to …"
- In the facial aesthetics presentation, two sections might be linked in this way: "So, I have shown you what the impact of sunshine is, so let's now consider ways to remove the wrinkles".

6.3.2.4   Ensure You Present Using Visual Elements Such as Previous Case Photos

The audience can easily lose focus if you simply talk at them and show endless amounts of data. Visual elements help to avoid this kind of monotonous delivery. Video clips serve a similar purpose [3, 6].

- Whenever possible, do not just tell your audience, but also show them through pre- and post-op photos. Visual understanding complements audio understanding.
- Try to find suitable short video clips. Having a different person explain the same issue also prevents the presentation from becoming too monotonous.
- Images are also very useful and usually should feature on the majority of slides.
- However, do not overplay your hand in terms of visual elements. Too heavy reliance on visuals may cause the audience to become confused or lose focus [2].

6.3.2.5   Concluding the Presentation

An effective conclusion draws together the whole presentation, relating the introduction to the ending and offering a brief summary of the main messages. The audience should be left still thinking about the material you covered. The concluding remarks should comprise no more than 5% or 10% of the total presentation. In other words, it should be succinct [6].

- A single slide should be enough for the conclusion. Remind the audience of the central message. Use a phrase, such as "So, as we have seen …" to signal you are summing up.
- The final slide could also be a visual if you have an infographic or diagram that encapsulates the central message.

6.3.3   Practising Delivery

Aim to present each slide for no longer than 1 or 2 min. Keep a note of how long it takes to present each section. Be aware that if you spend more than 2 min on a slide, your audience may show signs of boredom [6].

- If you need more time than this to present a slide, it is much better to reduce the information on each slide than to rush through presentation.
- To avoid speaking inaccurately, do not change the pace at which you would usually speak. Determine how much content to include by how much you can comfortably present within the allocated time.

Ensure the content has definite relevance to your message. Go through the presentation and remove any content which is irrelevant. Sometimes a fact or data may have been included because of interest but ask yourself whether such content is truly necessary to get the message across. Material should always be taken out of the presentation if it does not directly support the key message [3].

- Be aware, too, that you only need to present sufficient evidence to convince the audience of your point. It is tempting to aim to be comprehensive, but the old adage applies: "less is more".

Record How You Sound as You Present Listening to a recording of yourself presenting is a very practical and useful way to pick up areas of the delivery that require improvement [7].

- Adopt an enthusiastic tone whilst speaking. Avoid gaps in between sentences and use of "ergh …" or "umm …".
- Make sure that the transition between topics is smooth rather than abrupt. Use linking phrases to move from one point to the next.
- Keep a close eye on your timing. Avoid over-running. Audiences dislike presentations which over-run.
- If you practise in front of a mirror, you can pick up any tics or other movements that tend to distract the audience from what you are saying.

6.3.3.1 Continue to Practice Up to the Point Where Cue Cards Are Mostly Not Needed

Presenters who read from a script are typically less engaging than those who speak without notes. Small cards may be useful if they contain brief notes to jog your memory but aim to eliminate the need for notes as far as possible. With practice, you should reach a point where you can deliver without any awkward gaps where you need to refer to notes [4].

- Avoid simply reading the text contained on a diagram or graphic, as this makes the listeners lose engagement with the presentation.

6.4 Presentation Structure and Content

6.4.1 Content

In most cases, presenters start with a topic they are familiar with and have decided what they wish to say about it. This, then, will form the content of the presentation. Sometimes, a text already exists, which must then be presented. This may be the case when a report already exists in written form. However, whether the content needs to be composed de novo or is largely already determined, it will be necessary to shorten it to allow it to be presented. But why is this necessary?

- The main reason for shortening the content is the need to conform to the time limits on a presentation. This means presenters need to be selective about what content they include and choose only the most relevant material.
- The key indicator of success in a presentation is whether the audience remains engaged and attentive throughout the presentation. Presentations that are overloaded with material result in the audience losing focus by the end. Therefore, a presentation should be structured around the central messages, with material chosen to accomplish the communication of those messages.
- There are certain types of information which audiences typically struggle to understand fully during a presentation. This category includes highly technical information or large volumes of data. It may be better to present in a simpler way and refer the audience to reference documents they can consult after the presentation if they wish to obtain a fuller picture.
- Remember to allow space to give examples and present illustrations of any concepts you cover. Choose the examples carefully, so they offer maximum support and assistance in clarifying your argument.
- Furthermore, in any presentation, there is a need to introduce the topic at the beginning, draw a conclusion and allow questions or comments. Note that these elements have a degree of overlap with the main body of the presentation [8].

There are three factors which are especially worth considering when you are assembling content for a presentation, namely [8]:

- Which are the essential messages? Successful presentations rarely contain any more than five key messages.
- How can specific examples and illustrations be used most effectively to bolster the key messages?
- What will you do to allow the audience more easily to understand the key messages?

6.4.2   Structure

The majority of presentations are made up of introductory, main and concluding sections. Whilst the introduction serves to get the listeners ready to hear the points in the main section, the concluding section summarises and reiterates the messages of the main section. An effective presentation will increase the audience's interest in and curiosity about a subject. Skilled presenters welcome questions, not only at the end, but also during the presentation, and they are able to provide suitable replies [8].

6.4.2.1   Introductory Section

The introductory section achieves four main objectives, namely [8]:

- It gains the attention and focus of the listeners
- It lets the presenter speak, and the audience listen, comfortably
- It outlines why the presentation is being made and the objectives of the speaker
- It provides an outline of the main points that the presentation will cover

A good way to break the ice at the start of a presentation is to pose a question to the audience, tell a brief story, provide an interesting fact regarding the topic or showcase some unexpected visual element. It is quite common for presenters to then proceed onto a slide indicating the title, the objectives and the main outline of the presentation [8].

A story or a personal experience related to some current issue is a possible way to start a presentation, especially where the story or experience brings up important points to do with the main topic. A variant on this is to offer a short background or context to the current problem, leading to a brief formulation of the problem you wish to present about.

However you choose to begin, it is vital to make clear what your goal is in presenting. You can highlight the objective by saying something like [9]:

- *"Today's topic has become highly contentious, but I want to provide an overview of the issues involved"*
- *"By asking a particular question, we can work towards solutions …"*
- *"I will be arguing that …"*

In some cases, the presenter will need to narrow the focus to fit the time available. You might say [9]:

- *"Whilst there are numerous perspectives on the issue, I want to focus on the two I consider most productive, namely …"*
- *"The discussion will be confined to corporate waste, rather than recycling in general…"*
- *"Our focus today is on practical solutions, rather than business ethics …"*

Indicate to the audience how the presentation is structured [9]:

- *"There are three main themes to consider when talking about … first … then … and finally …"*

6.4.2.2 Body of the Presentation

The order in which you present the main body should be logical and appropriate to the topic, so that the audience can readily follow the argument. The material should be divided up into various sections which are clearly signposted to the audience. Pausing briefly when one section ends and before beginning the next is helpful. At this point, you might solicit questions, summarise what has been presented so far and highlight what you will cover next. It is possible to show the audience the outline of the talk, so they can follow where the presentation is going [8].

You can make the presentation more persuasive by adding specific illustrative examples and appropriate visuals. When doing so, bear in mind the following questions [8]:

- Does the example reflect what the audience has already experienced?
- Is the example concrete enough?
- Are the examples interesting by themselves?
- Is there enough variety in the examples chosen?
- Will the audience remember the examples afterwards?

The body is where you showcase the evidence to support your argument or thesis. Each of the main messages should be explained clearly and coherently. Ensure that the relationship between the points you are making is comprehensible and that the points help advance your argument [9]. You can help the audience to understand by using phrases such as:

- *"Moving on to our next point …"*
- *"A further matter to consider is …"*
- *"Now we have looked at this issue, there is another point I would like to discuss …"*

Whenever you introduce a new concept or unfamiliar term, remember to supply a definition and explanation of what is meant. Tie in the examples that you are using as illustrations [9].

6.4.2.3   The Final Stage: Concluding

An effective conclusion accomplishes two tasks, namely [8]:

- It reiterates the salient messages from the presentation
- It strengthens the key central theme

Always end positively, on an upbeat note. The audience should have the feeling that they gained something valuable by listening to the presentation [8].

Once you reach the end of your material, make it clear by saying something like:

- *"Thus, in conclusion …"*
- *"Let me finish by stating …"*

Remember to provide a succinct summary whilst concluding. You can reiterate why the topic is so important, restate the learning objective(s) and show how the presentation addressed these objectives. End by expressing gratitude to the audience for listening to you and signal that you would like to hear any questions or comments they have [9].

6.4.2.4 Dealing with Questions

It is common for presenters to be concerned about questions that may be asked in a presentation. Nonetheless, the fact that audience members are asking questions signals that they have been engaging with the topic. A lack of questions is actually an indicator that the presentation may not have fully succeeded. You can direct the types of questions you would like the audience to ask by highlighting possible points that call for clarification. Furthermore, if you leave some pauses between sections and address questions as they come up, the whole process may be smoother. Although questions do add a much-needed element of interactivity, be wary of spending too long on answering them. If necessary, indicate that you will address more complex questions at the end. Once you have addressed the questions at pauses during the presentation, you need to rapidly move on with the rest of the presentation to avoid losing momentum [8].

6.4.2.5 Avoiding Plagiarism

As with any publication, where you rely on other people's ideas or use an image they created, this needs to receive acknowledgement in the form of a reference. Sometimes this will be written on a slide, at other times the presenter may say the reference. Make sure that references do not interfere with the flow of any text. It is quite acceptable to list all the references on one of the final slides of the presentation [9].

References

1. Giving Presentations. https://columbiacollege-ca.libguides.com/presentations/planning. Accessed 4 Oct 2021.
2. Taylor C. How to plan a presentation. Last Updated: Mar 29, 2019. https://www.wikihow.com/Plan-a-Presentation. Accessed 4 Oct 2021.
3. http://www.garrreynolds.com/preso-tips/prepare/.
4. http://tutorials.istudy.psu.edu/oralpresentations/oralpresentations3.html.
5. http://www2.le.ac.uk/offices/ld/resources/presentations/planning-presentation.
6. http://stemdiv.ucsc.edu/files/4513/1717/0253/OralPresentationHO_2007.pdf.
7. https://www.nottingham.ac.uk/studyingeffectively/preparing/presentations/delivering.aspx.
8. Oral presentation—content and structure. http://www4.caes.hku.hk/epc/presentation/content_and_structure.asp. Accessed 4 Oct 2021.
9. Structuring your presentation. Australian National University. https://www.anu.edu.au/students/academic-skills/writing-assessment/presentations/structuring-your-presentation.

7.1   Introduction

Although these days meetings can occur in many different formats, one constant is the need to make a favourable first impression.

The first impression you create has an enormous impact on business performance, as it largely determines what ideas potential clients may subsequently form about you and your products or services. Some factors to consider include:

- Do you create an impression of friendliness, being knowledgeable and ready to help?
- Does the impression you convey lead clients to feel that you can be relied on to act in their best interests?

A favourable initial impression opens the way to a fruitful business relationship, whereas a negative initial impression may place hurdles in the way of doing business that prove impossible to overcome.

Since many initial meetings now occur online, there is a need to understand how to come across well in virtual meetings. This is the subject of the current chapter, which covers the best techniques to use.

There are ways in which initial meetings over videoconference (such as Zoom) can equal or even surpass face-to-face (F2F) meetings as an opportunity to establish a favourable first impression [1], as will be discussed here.

7.2   Tips on Creating a Favourable Initial Impression

7.2.1   Dress as You Normally Would for Business

Whilst there is an understandable temptation to dress down when business is being conducted from your home office with you sitting at the keyboard all day, this is not an ideal way to create a positive impression. Clothes that are stained and frayed convey the impression that you are not taking business fully seriously.

Conversely, unless the meeting would usually require you to dress in formal attire, there is no need to do this online. In most business contexts it is acceptable to dress in smart casual clothing, such as a shirt with a collar or a plain jumper. This style of clothing makes you appear to be serious about the meeting but does not draw too much attention to your appearance.

Personal grooming is also a key factor to consider. Make sure you look well-groomed and tidy. The very first thing any client will notice about you is your general appearance and if you appear "under the weather", a client may make a snap judgement that your performance will be similarly less than perfect [1].

7.2.2   Ensure the Background Is Suitable

In F2F meetings, formal or otherwise, it is rarely necessary to consider in detail what the room behind you looks like. With videoconferenced meetings, however, the backdrop assumes far greater importance, and this is something that you will definitely have to pay attention to.

Ideally, present from a location that has a plain-looking background. If there is light coming from outside, that is ideal. However, if such a space is unavailable, there is the option on Zoom to use a virtual background. The application has several backgrounds already installed, or they can be found online at no cost. The background can then be attached to the user profile and displayed at the next meeting. The following steps indicate how to do this on Zoom [1]:

- Log in to the Zoom website at the following address: www.zoom.us.
- Choose the "settings" menu from the options displayed on the left of the screen.
- Select "In Meeting (Advanced)".
- Go down the list that comes up until you encounter "virtual background", which should be enabled.
- Now launch the Zoom desktop application on your device, making sure you log in.
- There should be an icon which resembles a cogwheel. It is at the top right-hand corner of the screen.
- Choose "virtual background".
- You can then select from one of the pre-existing backgrounds or upload either an image or video to use as a custom background. Clicking on the plus side lets you do this.

Consider also how you will be illuminated on the screen. Whenever possible, make use of natural lighting. If that is not possible (for example, when there is no window), make sure at least that the main source of illumination does not leave you in shadow, such as when the main light is coming from behind you [1].

7.2.3   Look Towards the Camera Whilst Speaking

It is common for people on a teleconference to look at the screen but bear in mind that you should look towards wherever the camera is when speaking, so as to convey a better impression.

In many cases, the camera involved will be the webcam built into your laptop. Although the screen and camera are in the same general direction, if you are looking at the screen, you are not actually reproducing the eye contact that normally occurs in such a setting. Looking towards the camera will help to reduce this sense of artificiality in the meeting.

Making eye contact is an integral part of communication when it occurs F2F. Being able to look someone in the eye whilst they are speaking not only gives the impression that person is being honest with you, but also sends a clear signal that the focus is on you.

Thus, eye contact is something you should always strive to achieve if you want to make a favourable first impression on someone.

Accordingly, in a Zoom meeting, if you look into the camera, rather than at the screen, as you are talking, you will give the other person the feeling you are making eye contact, which will undoubtedly add considerably to a favourable impression [1].

7.2.3.1   Keep the Cameras Rolling

If the meeting occurs in a format where having your camera on is permitted, switch the camera on. Being able to see each other typically makes participants more engaged and lets the others get to know you more easily. In situations where the camera needs to remain switched off for any reason, it is important to maintain interactivity in other ways, so that everybody present knows that the other meeting participants are still actively engaged and interested. This can be achieved through chat messaging, polls, etc.

7.2.3.2   Think About Where the Light Comes From

The best way to illuminate your face is by lighting coming from the front. An ideal situation is where light from a window falls on your face. Alternatively, a lamp positioned to light your face also works well. Light coming from above also provides satisfactory illumination. However, a light source behind the speaker will cast the face into shadow and makes it hard for others to see you on the screen [2].

7.2.3.3 Establish Good Camera Angles

To make sure the camera on a laptop computer or mobile phone is at the right level, the device may need to be propped up on a purpose-designed stand or an improvised stand, such as a pile of books. Just ensure that the camera angle does not mean cutting off half your face or staring up at your face from an unflattering angle [2].

7.2.3.4 Show a Clean-Looking Background

Just as you would not want to appear in a business meeting wearing a string vest, so it is worth considering the background, since anything in the background may appear on screen. The kind of embarrassing item you do not want to appear are things like racy posters or pin-ups, dirty washing, another inhabitant of your home or private items.

If all else fails, and there is no suitable location from which to join a meeting, some videoconferencing applications, such as Zoom, do offer virtual backgrounds. It is important, however, not to choose a background that is distracting to other meeting participants [2].

7.2.3.5 Look Towards the Camera

Many people who are attending a teleconference tend to watch the screen rather than looking into the camera. Whilst it is easy to understand that participants want to check how others, or they themselves, appear on camera, it has the unfortunate effect that it may seem the participant is looking elsewhere or is not fully engaged. By consciously looking into the camera, both whilst speaking and whilst listening, you can convey the impression that you are making eye contact and thus appear to be actively participating.

If there is any reason why you cannot have your camera switched on, at least if you upload a picture of yourself to your profile, it gives a visual reminder to the other meeting attendees that you are present [2].

7.2.4 Muting the Microphone

The widespread adoption of videoconferencing, especially following the COVID-19 pandemic, has meant many people unexpectedly began working or studying from home. In such circumstances, meetings or presentations frequently get interrupted by unexpected sounds, like dogs barking, ambulances passing or children shouting.

Whilst few people are greatly shocked by such interruptions, it is still greatly preferable to avoid such interruptions as much as possible. The mute feature on the microphone is an important tool to keep unexpected interruptions from occurring.

The first precaution to take, however, is to join the meeting from an environment which is as quiet as possible. Whenever you are not speaking yourself, you can mute your microphone, which prevents noise being picked up. On Zoom, keeping the space bar depressed unmutes the microphone. When you release the space bar, the mute is reapplied. This feature is helpful for when you want to give a short reply, for instance.

Of course, being in a noisy environment also makes listening to another person more difficult. In a meeting, you may easily miss a vital piece of information. Furthermore, if the other party notes that you were not fully listening, this may leave an unfavourable impression about your professional approach [1].

Participants in a videoconference should show that they are interested and engaged in the proceedings. When the participants communicate these positive feelings, the atmosphere in the virtual meeting is more conducive to learning and contributing. Presenters communicating positive engagement facilitate contributions from individuals who may be less outgoing but still have important questions to ask [2].

Be aware, too, that certain actions that people commonly perform at home may convey a disrespectful attitude when seen online, for example, glancing repeatedly at your watch, checking your mobile device, eating or playing with a pet animal. It is also generally better not to get up and move around, once a presentation or meeting has begun [2].

7.2.4.1 If the Connection Slows Down, Switch Off the Video Feed

Signs of a slow internet connection include problems with the audio signal, a pixelated appearance on video, "unstable connection" warnings or freezing. A limitation on bandwidth can be partly overcome by switching off the video feed, although, generally speaking, most people do prefer to be able to see the other people involved in communication. If the video feed does need to be cut, it is better if you have a picture of yourself to accompany your profile, so that there is a visible reminder of who you are, rather than just have a black screen with a username appear [2].

7.2.5 Video Is Not the Same as F2F

It is much more challenging for someone to understand body language from the view typically captured by a webcam than by seeing someone F2F. This relates to the fact that the webcam only captures the front view of the head and upper torso. When speaking in this situation, you should make any gestures that accompany your words within the field of view of the camera.

Conversely, there are some actions which participants in videoconferences need to make sure are not captured by video, as these actions tend to make a less favourable impression. Examples include eating or letting your eyes wander away from the screen.

Indeed, to make the most favourable impression, whether F2F or virtually, there is one simple rule: show that you are interested in the conversation and engaged in the discussion. To achieve this impression online, make sure you have the right camera angle, remove things that may distract you and ensure your focus is clearly on the meeting you are attending.

It ought to go without saying that a friendly smile is also a big asset in making a favourable impression.

7.2.6   Have the Right Appearance

Whilst it is true that making a snap judgement on someone based on his or her appearance is an unwise thing to do, the fact remains that a neatly presented, well-dressed presenter has a definitely higher chance of making a favourable first impression than one in soiled clothing who appears to have just crawled out of bed. This is an unfortunate fact of life. Furthermore, not only do others rate you more highly when you make an effort to appear smart, but it also boosts your own confidence when speaking. You can be more relaxed, knowing that a smart appearance already begins to affect the audience positively before you utter the first word [3].

7.2.7   Pay Attention to Your Body Language

Being appropriately dressed is, however, unlikely to positively influence an audience if your body language contradicts the first impression. Avoid slouching in your chair or failing to smile. Actions like crossing the arms in front of your chest or biting your lips convey the impression that you are a defensive, or even aggressive, individual.

So, before speaking, whether F2F or online, spend a little time attending to your own body language and relaxing your facial muscles into a smile. Audiences will remember a friendly looking and relaxed presenter much more positively than one who looked totally stressed-out and anxious at the thought of speaking [3].

7.2.8   Make Sure You Feel Comfortable First

In the majority of cases, presenters who are uncomfortable in some way (perhaps because their outfit is scratchy, the shoes pinch or they are aware of poor self-grooming) give out unconscious signals about the discomfort that the audience easily pick up on. To avoid sending out such messages, choose an outfit that is comfortable to wear and choose shoes that fit. Having fewer external distractions means you will achieve a much sharper focus on delivering the key message of your presentation [3].

7.2.9   Develop Mastery in Communication

For many individuals, having the confidence to give a presentation at an important meeting or be the main speaker at a conference is not something that comes naturally. However, if you work on your communication skills, you both make a favourable impression and can deliver a more effective presentation. Use a mirror to practise your delivery and make sure the material becomes familiar enough that you can present it easily and without hesitation [3].

7.2.10 Accentuate the Positivity

People who appear cheerful convey the impression they are more charismatic, trustworthy and fun to be with. By accentuating the positive, you first sell yourself as a presenter before you sell the message of the presentation. Being positive and upbeat is vital to making a favourable first impression. Sales representatives who convey gloom and boredom are unlikely to convince anyone to buy.

The first impression is formed very quickly, within seconds of first meeting someone. This initial impression then strongly influences how far someone will trust you and focus on what you have to say. Ask yourself these questions, to assess how you appear and sound to others:

Are you conveying a smart and hygienic appearance?
Are you pronouncing words clearly and distinctly?
Are you generally smiling and acting in a natural way?

Having learnt how best to mould first impressions about you favourably, you will have an enduring advantage in terms of convincing any audience and getting them to follow your presentation.

Therefore, before presenting, always ask yourself what kind of first impression you are making. Everything else depends on that.

References

1. A good business presentation starts strong. https://www.effectivepresentations.com/blog/make-a-good-first-impression-on-zoom/. Accessed 4 Oct 2021.
2. Tips for making a good impression in virtual meetings. The University of Southern Mississippi. https://www.usm.edu/student-success/tips-virtual-meetings.php. Accessed 4 Oct 2021.
3. The importance of first impressions. https://www.effectivepresentations.com/blog/win-over-your-audience-with-a-good-first-impression/. Accessed 4 Oct 2021.

Analysing Your Audience in Advance 8

8.1 Introduction

Audience analysis is a concept of increasing prominence in the fields of business and public speaking. One of the key reasons for a presentation to fail is because the audience is unable to focus on the topic, or there is an apparent lack of interest in the topic. The key to resolving this type of problem is to conduct a thorough audience analysis before presenting.

For too long, many presenters have overlooked the central importance of the audience in the success or failure of a presentation. However audience analysis has now become an integral part of preparing a presentation. Just as the great orators and public speakers of the past were able to find the common interests that united large groups of individuals, in spite of their different viewpoints and attitudes, so any presenter must aim to find what the audience members have in common.

This chapter details the step-by-step process needed to analyse an audience. Audience analysis lets the presenter establish stronger rapport and present more efficiently and persuasively [1].

8.2 What Does "Audience Analysis" Mean?

In any type of communicative exchange, communication is more effective when the parties involved know something about each other's background. The term "audience analysis" denotes research carried out on the audience for a presentation, from which conclusions can be drawn about how best to present. Whenever a presentation is given, the audience plays a major role, and being able to tailor a presentation to suit an audience is an indicator of a highly skilled presenter.

Making rapid judgements about a new acquaintance can be fraught with risk. However, some of the techniques used in audience analysis can provide clues about

C. C. Cingi et al., *Improving Online Presentations*,
https://doi.org/10.1007/978-3-031-28328-4_8

what another person may be expecting. This chapter will address audience analysis methods that are of value in preparing both one-to-one and one-to-many presentations [1].

8.3   What Is the Importance of Analysing an Audience?

8.3.1   Understanding an Audience Is Helpful in Setting the Right Tone and Building Trust

Knowing what expectations your audience has facilitates stronger connections based on meeting those expectations. For communication to occur with the highest level of efficiency, there needs to be a significant degree of overlap between what the speaker suggests and what the audience can accept between recommended courses of action and probable audience response. The deeper a presenter understands the audience, the greater the likelihood of mutual benefit. If you can offer realistic solutions to problems that are causing an audience pain, they will be more likely to trust you.

8.3.2   Understanding How an Audience Tends to React Lets You Craft More Persuasive Calls to Action

If you comprehend the value system of your intended listeners, you will better understand their decision-making. Such knowledge is a vital asset in spotting unexpected opportunities to do business or work together on projects, with different individuals. Whether a presentation is primarily educational in nature, or is designed to pitch for sales, an appreciation of how audiences react provides speakers with a competitive edge. You should understand whether an audience is driven by considerations of economy (financial or effort), or whether achieving the best possible result is the motivator. By referring to your audience's expectations, you make the presentation more hard-hitting.

8.3.3   Presentations Should Be Modified so that the Key Messages Align with the Audience's Requirements and Expectations

Through understanding your audience, you can predict what sort of response will occur to different sections of the presentation. Analysis of an audience provides insight into their emotional triggers, the levers of persuasion and the areas where offence may occur. It can translate into a list of things to include or exclude from a presentation. Furthermore, the presenter can decide on the most effective tone to adopt, what sort of examples and explanations to provide, when to inject humour and how to urge the audience into action. A well-tailored presentation of this kind achieves the greatest impact [1].

8.4   The Advantages of Knowing Your Audience

By presenting, you are aiming at educating your audience and getting them to approve of what you are telling them. By "audience" is meant anything from a single individual through to a giant public meeting. Furthermore, audiences may be present face-to-face or online (i.e. virtually). An audience may be restricted to a few chosen people or may be open to anyone interested. One virtually invariable feature of presentations is, however, that the presenter speaks for significantly longer than the audience. The audience tend to spend most of their time in the listener role. When there is little in the way of audience interaction, either questions or feedback, there exists an imbalance in the communicative roles. This balance may be altered when members of the audience pose questions or provide feedback by commenting or giving applause [2].

8.4.1   Presenting in an Audience-Centric Way

The fact that communication is imbalanced in this way means that presenters rarely have the chance to go over material a second or third time after realising that the message has not been effectively delivered. Thus, when a presentation is being prepared, understanding your audience is the best way to make sure the message can be understood at first hearing. Presentations that conform to this approach may be termed "audience-centric".

When delivering a presentation to a group, it is the audience that you are addressing and on whose behalf you are speaking. This allows us to appreciate the centrality of the audience in presenting. Indeed, being familiar with the audience is amongst the key tasks involved. It is important to find out as much as possible about the audience demographics—age group, gender, level of education, religious affiliation and cultural values. You need to know what groups your audience are members of. If you can understand what your audience believes, how they see certain issues and what they value, you can predict their reactions and target the message more accurately [2].

8.4.2   Establishing Mutual Interests by Understanding Others' Viewpoints

Audience analysis is part of the preparation phase of presentation. Its purpose is to allow the presenter to establish a connection with the audience. The process involves putting yourself in the audience's shoes and attempting to see issues the way they would. This exercise helps to establish what mutual interest presenters and the audience share and means the presenter can shape the message delivered so that it is in harmony with the audience's pre-existing knowledge and beliefs [2].

8.4.3   Discovering and Collating Information on the Audience

Audience analysis refers to the collation and analysis of information about any audience, whether the intended communication is spoken, written or visual. The techniques involved range from the most basic, for example, simply asking a representative group about what they already know and believe, through to more complex analysis of demographic research carried out on similar groups to the one that will constitute the audience. Analysis can be carried out by using surveys (possibly including rating scales) which ask about demographic details and attitudes. Although there are many other techniques which might be employed, the key feature any technique must have is that it provides the information needed to craft the most effective presentation. When the data have been analysed, it should be possible to construct a profile of the audience members, which will provide insights into the best way to communicate to maximise delivery of the message [2].

8.4.4   How Audience Analysis Really Helps Presenters

Knowing these details about the intended audience lets you prepare a message that is optimised in terms of intelligibility and relevance. There are two areas, in particular, where audience analysis has an especially practical relevance: to avoid saying things which may alienate the audience, such as ill-judged humour, and to speak at the most appropriate level for the audience, so they find the presentation easy to grasp and relevant to their interests. A presentation that comes across to the audience as informative and engaging has a far greater chance of succeeding [2].

8.5   What Should You Analyse?

Analysis of an audience includes establishing the following about them: the age structure, gender balance, sexual orientation, degree of education, religious affiliation, cultural factors, race and ethnicity [2].

8.5.1   First Examine Your Own Biases

Presenters need first to try to uncover their own prejudices and biases, which can prevent them from seeing the world through another person's eyes. Examine what you believe, what your attitudes usually are and what you hold valuable. When you question your own biases, it is easier to put yourself in the audience's shoes and appreciate how they tend to view the world.

Presenters who fail to engage in this process of self-questioning are at risk of becoming ego-centric. Ego-centric individuals cannot grasp what others truly think, since they consider their own attitudes, beliefs and thoughts to be the only reasonable ones to hold. This ego-centric perspective then blinds such individuals to how others perceive and means they fail to appreciate that another person's reality is quite different from their own and equally valid [2].

8.5.2   Comprehending the Background Factors, Attitudes and Beliefs of Audiences

Successful presenters need to know who they are presenting to, where they come from and the way they tend to think. However, this information needs to be gathered in as time-efficient and effective a way as possible. One part of audience analysis that can usually be gathered efficiently is the demographic characteristics. A demographic analysis involves statistical treatment of the data gathered about specific features of a human population.

When performing the demographics portion of an audience analysis, a sociological approach is generally the most fruitful. In other words, the following are the questions presenters need to answer:

- Does the audience consist of all men, all women or a mixed group?
- Does the group have shared experiences?
- Is it a group defined by sexual orientation?
- What level of education do they have?
- Are they all of the same religious affiliation?
- What is their culture, race and ethnicity?

Besides these demographic particulars, the analysis should also delve into the characteristic attitudes and beliefs of the audience. Think about how the audience views particular individuals, events or ideas. The attitudes an audience may hold may range from extreme hostility towards welcoming acceptance. Alternatively, they may be ambivalent about some issues or hold no fixed opinions at all. Presenters benefit from knowing about the views that audience members are likely to already have as this allows them to adapt the presentation so that it harmonises with pre-existing beliefs to the maximum possible extent. The arguments of a presentation can be rendered more convincing if this knowledge of attitudes is applied [2].

8.5.3   Advice for Presenters

The number of individuals expected in the audience and the way the presentation is to be delivered both have a bearing on how extensive the audience analysis is, as well as how it is undertaken. If there will only be a few attendees, and the event is F2F, it may be adequate just to speak with them prior to the presentation. Nonetheless, if there are expected to be more people in the audience, or the presentation is virtual, sending a survey or questionnaire to fill out prior to the event may be a more practical strategy to employ [2].

8.6   How Can You Assess Your Audience?

Hopefully by now you have been convinced of the value of carrying out an audience analysis when preparing a presentation. However, there is still the difficulty of how to actually carry out the analysis on a group of unfamiliar individuals. The following factors are worth taking a note of, since they are reliable indicators of an audience's true characteristics [1].

8.6.1   Demographic Characteristics

Demographic characteristics include items such as age distribution, gender, education level, profession or job, ethnic identity, financial situation and relationship status. This information is suitable for statistical analysis. How old the audience are and the extent of their education are of especial interest, as these factors determine the level of the presentation. If you overestimate the ability of the audience to understand the material, the presentation may leave them feeling confused, whereas underestimating their level of comprehension may lead to a presentation perceived as boring or even patronising. Audiences with different backgrounds will bring different interests to the presentation. Armed with this information, the presentation can be adjusted to suit the audience.

8.6.2   Pre-existing Knowledge About a Topic

It is essential to determine what your audience already knows about a subject. This will then inform how you begin the presentation. When presenting to novices or non-specialists, there may need to be an introduction to the topic and an explanation of its importance. This is required to stimulate the audience's interest. However, if addressing professionals or specialists, this part may be omitted as they already appreciate the significance of the topic. Thus, if you are informed about what your audience already knows, you may be able to shorten the material and make it easier to present. Furthermore, the presenter can choose the appropriate degree of technical language to include in the presentation.

8.6.3   The Number of Attendees and the Venue

The method of delivery varies considerably, according to audience size. A classroom with a dozen students is quite different from a business conference with several 100 delegates in attendance. Likewise, the tone depends on the occasion. An after dinner speaker at a Rotary Club event will be more humorous than someone delivering a eulogy at a funeral. The size of the expected audience also influences the possibilities for interaction. Interacting with five people is very different from interacting with 500.

The venue is also a key factor. Compare a private meeting room with a village hall. It is important to know what kind of equipment may be used. Can you project slides or would a speech be a more appropriate format?

The time of the presentation also has an impact on how the audience will react. Every speaker can sense when they have been given the "graveyard slot" when the audience is least liable to stay awake for the presentation.

8.6.4 Audience's Value Systems and Beliefs

The degree of openness amongst audiences towards new concepts or ideas is very much influenced by their religious beliefs, culture and upbringing. For some individuals, any new belief can only be accepted insofar as it fits in with their existing beliefs. An audience may, however, contain individuals with extremely varied outlooks and values, in which case the most that can probably be achieved is to present without provoking an ideological conflict in the minds of those present.

8.6.5 How Does the Audience Normally Receive Information?

Think about the usual way the audience receive new information. For example, are they more focused on online sources or printed material? Have there been similar presentations to yours, which the audience have attended for updates? Do they know the subject matter experts or have direct involvement in research themselves? The answers to these questions have a bearing in deciding the format of the presentation. If you have an audience that is used to debate, you will need thought-provoking activities. Conversely, audiences who prefer bite-size information may benefit more from brief thumbnail sketches and summaries.

8.7 Ways to Deal with Various Types of Audience

As we have discussed, audiences differ in the way they respond, due to the fundamental differences between them. The following sections define some common scenarios and outline advice on how to deal with each.

An audience may consist of individuals who do not readily alter their opinions and powerful reasoning may be needed to persuade them to adopt a fresh viewpoint. Conversely, if you are addressing individuals who have already volunteered to undertake a particular task, convincing them may be extremely straightforward. Another type of audience contains key opinion leaders (KOLs). If you bring the KOLs onboard, the others tend to fall in line with the new viewpoint. KOLs then make sure the message translates into action [1].

8.7.1 The Hostile Audience: Sceptical Individuals, Who Need Hard Evidence

Hostile individuals in the audience at a presentation tend to be rather ego-centric. They believe their own opinions must be correct. If there are many such individuals present, the audience will be less willing to consider novel ideas and ways of seeing a problem. Although this scenario can feel alarming, keep calm, as there are ways to deal with it.

Let the hostile audience members express their view and ensure you emphasise those viewpoints you do have in common. Being listened to is what ego-centric individuals generally crave. However, avoid distorting your claims just to fit what such people want. Focus on providing clear and specific evidence to support your viewpoint and remember to express your conclusions in a confident way.

8.7.2 The Welcoming Audience: Build on Natural Rapport to Get the Message Across

Some audiences are already enthusiastic about the subject of the presentation and ready to hear whatever you can tell them. They respond positively to the presentation and agree with the viewpoint you advance.

For such audiences, speak in a passionate way and work with their emotions through giving examples that speak most strongly to them. The welcoming audience is the one most likely to stick with your idea. They are readily persuaded. In such a circumstance, make sure you give a clear indication what action you want or what message they need to take onboard, whether that is signing a sales contract or adjusting professional practice in some way.

8.7.3 The Apathetic Audience: You Have to Persuade Them That the Topic Really Matters

Apathetic audiences consist of people who have little or no interest in the subject you are presenting. They neither agree nor disagree but are mostly just wanting to get on with something else. It is likely they will be distracted easily during the presentation.

The initial approach to such an audience is to draw them into the discussion. Pose simple questions and listen patiently to their responses. Make use of attention-grabbing visuals and note how they respond. Build a strong case point by point, emphasising why it is relevant to them as individuals. Rather than showcasing your own expertise, concentrate on convincing these people that they have something to gain from the topic.

8.7.4   The Uninformed Audience: Individuals Who Are New to the Subject

Uninformed audiences are those where the audience members have little prior knowledge of the subject. It is possible they have a basic understanding, but not more. They are attending because they want to have a deeper knowledge. Their expectation is that the presenter will guide them through the basics.

Accordingly, before going straight into the details, check what the audience already know and move steadily from the fundamentals, emphasising how to apply the new knowledge. Do not try to get your audience to act before you have provided them with a firm knowledge base. It is especially important not to overwhelm your audience with technical terms and language at this point, as they may become confused.

In the majority of cases, an audience will contain several different types of individuals. Presenters require the flexibility to adapt presentations according to the needs of different audience members.

8.8   Application of the Information Gathered by Audience Analysis

Suppose that you have carried out a full analysis of your audience and can predict the audience's expectations. How should this information be used to prepare or modify the presentation? Where will you make adjustments? After all, the whole purpose of performing the analysis is to be able to improve the effectiveness of the presentation. The following sections indicate how you can apply the insights gained by audience analysis.

8.8.1   Remember to Present in an Audience-Centric Way

Never forget that the audience are central to any presentation. Let the audience know how they will benefit from your presentation. Indeed, check with them what their expectations actually are. When you tell an audience about a new idea, show them how the idea relates to their experience. When you want to showcase a product, it is better to emphasise how it will help the client than to list all the product's features. Or if you need to present the results of a research project, relate the findings to the current state of knowledge and what the practical implications are. Ensure that examples you select will resonate with the audience.

8.8.2   Establish Mutual Interests

Individuals always differ in how they see the world and in their underlying beliefs, thus no presentation can ever precisely tell the audience what they want to know in the precise manner in which they want to hear it. This may be an unattainable ideal, but there are still many advantages to identifying where the mutual interests of the presenter and the audience members lie. Do not try to be a version of the audience members themselves, as this would appear fake. Conversely, being overly dogmatic and insistent that your views are the only valid ones come across as aggressive and arrogant. Try to achieve a balance, which will then mean the presentation works for different kinds of audience.

8.8.3 Construct a Typical Audience Persona and Practise Addressing the Persona

Construct a persona that represents a typical member of your intended audience, based on the information you have assembled in the audience analysis. When practising, imagine the persona is listening. People want to feel that they are important and have your complete attention. Try to speak so they feel you are personally addressing them. The persona helps presenters to tailor their approach with the demographic details and characteristic beliefs and expectations of the audience firmly in mind. Not only is this technique of value in formal presentations, it can also be used for sales pitches or other occasions when you address an audience.

8.8.4 Know Where the Audience Pain Points Are and Acknowledge Them Whilst Presenting

With the audience's pain points and their expectations clearly in view, presenters can plan the best way to approach the topic. Acknowledge the issues audience members have and offer potential resolutions. Let them see how the service or product you are advocating has the potential to improve matters. Make use of analytical tools, such as Google analytics, to find out what queries members of the public ask about a topic. If the presentation has clearly led the audience to the idea that the product, service or approach you are recommending is the solution to their problems, it will have achieved the maximum possible impact. The presentation then naturally leads to the call for action you wish to make.

8.8.5 When Necessary, Segment Your Audience

If it seems more feasible to segment the audience and present in a different way to different groups, be prepared to act accordingly. Some topics are of greater relevance to certain groups than others. The audience analysis may reveal the best way to segment the audience into groups. The advantages of segmentation are both to the presenter and the audience members. The presenter can retain a straightforward approach, unhindered by trying to address disparate requirements, and the audience faces a presentation more exactly matching their needs.

References

1. Bharat P. Audience analysis for presentations: how to know your audience and present better. 2018. https://slidebazaar.com/blog/audience-analysis-in-presentations/. Accessed 4 Oct 2021.
2. The importance of audience analysis https://courses.lumenlearning.com/boundless-communications/chapter/the-importance-of-audience-analysis/. Accessed 4 Oct 2021.

Interacting with Your Virtual Audience

9

9.1 Introduction

If you prepare a presentation to deliver online without considering how to engage the audience, your presentation will be missing an absolutely essential component. Indeed, by incorporating audience engagement as a core element, you ensure the effectiveness and memorability of the presentation will be maximised.

Fortunately, there exist multiple methods for keeping an audience engaged as they view a presentation online. Presenters need to consider carefully the objectives in presenting together with the intended audience and can deploy several special techniques that apply to the virtual arena [1].

9.2 What Form Do You Want Audience Engagement to Take?

One of the first matters to consider is the way your presentation will unfold and the form of engagement you want from your audience. There are certain questions to ask, the answers to which will then lead you towards the best engagement method to utilise. Such questions include:

- What kind of information will the audience be asked to provide?
- How does the presenter intend to use this information?
- What level of interaction between audience members themselves will occur during the presentation?
- Are there individuals within the audience who can provide information of importance to the audience as a whole?
- What are the reasons for the audience to attend? What sort of learning objectives do they have? Do they wish to contribute their own experience? What sort of queries are they likely to have? [1]

© The Author(s), under exclusive license to Springer Nature
Switzerland AG 2023
C. C. Cingi et al., *Improving Online Presentations*,
https://doi.org/10.1007/978-3-031-28328-4_9

9.3   Techniques for Maintaining Audience Engagement

9.3.1   First Technique: Polling

Polling is a useful technique to gather responses from an audience. Polling capabilities are built into several videoconferencing applications or exist as standalone solutions. Information gathered can be in the form of a constricted choice (such as a multiple choice question (MCQ)) or may allow for a freer response. The results of the poll are immediately visible to the presenter, who can make a decision whether to share the result immediately, store it for later use or highlight features of it to the audience [1].

Polling is designed to achieve two principal goals [1]:

9.3.1.1   To Gather Information from the Audience

Some examples of situations where a poll may be used to gather information from the attendees at a presentation are as follows:

- To check the existing level of knowledge an audience has about a subject, so that the content of the presentation can be adjusted to suit them.
- A chance for the audience to feed back. This may occur between presentations, for example.
- Yes/no or MCQ type questions at regular intervals during a presentation, to give the presenter feedback on how effectively the message is being delivered.
- To create a word cloud, made up of responses from the audience, and summarising their collective opinions, emotions or thoughts in a readily understood format with high aesthetic appeal.

Using polls in this way keeps the audience engaged whilst also giving the presenter valuable feedback on which to act.

9.3.1.2   For Engagement, but Also to Let the Audience Interact with Each Other

If the aim of the poll is less about gathering information and more about maximising how engaged your audience is, the following ways of using a poll may be suitable:

- Posing a challenging, interesting or unexpected question, especially in a keynote speech.
- Setting up a fastest on the button competition, with a leaderboard, to make the event more exciting.
- As an icebreaker, where you want the audience members to reveal an interesting fact about themselves.

General advice on how best to use polls [1]:

- It is a good idea to include a poll whenever you present.

- In a presentation lasting for 1 h, the frequency of polling should be at least each quarter of an hour. In half-hour sessions, the frequency is even higher, say every 6 or 7 min.
- If it is feasible, pose up to 3 audience survey questions at a time, so that the audience really engages with the topic.
- When you first set up the event and invite participants, remember to include a poll question. You could also get the audience members to try out the poll before the main presentations at a conference. That way, the audience already understands what will be required when a survey question comes up.
- It may be useful also to set up poll questions to occur at various points so that you can check the audience are still actively listening to the presentation, rather than being logged on but currently engaged in some other activity.

9.3.2 Second Technique: Questions and Answers (Q&As)

There are many different ways to set up Q&As in a presentation. The following are some of the methods available [1]:

9.3.2.1 Open Format Q&A

Open Format via Audio With this method, you let the attendees interrupt the session by speaking. They can unmute their own microphones. This technique is best suited to situations where there are few attendees and perhaps they already know each other, such as a group of colleagues.

Chat Functionality If you enable the chat function, the audience members can ask questions by writing them in the chat. Either the presenters themselves, or event managers, can screen the questions submitted via chat and choose the best ones for the presenter to answer.

Chat can also be set up in such a way that it allows a conversation to flow during the presentation. A moderator is generally required. The audience can interact with each other, rather than simply asking questions to the presenter. The moderator may direct the conversation by asking for opinions on themes raised by the presentation or may highlight important messages from the talk to stimulate a response.

9.3.2.2 Specific Time for Q&A

Allocating a specific time for Q&A (typically at the end of a presentation) may be the most appropriate method if there are large numbers of attendees or the topic needs to be presented without gaps in the delivery. It is best to have already assembled a few questions before the presentation finishes, so that there is no inconvenient wait before questions begin to arrive.

One way to combine setting specific times for Q&A with a greater level of interaction is to space Q&A throughout the presentation at regular intervals, such as every quarter of an hour. This method has the advantage of increasing audience interest and engagement. Not only is it more interactive, but it also means that questions relate to the material just presented. The presenter may answer in such a way as to naturally lead into the following sections of the presentation.

Another possibility is to ask for questions even before the presentation or conference actually takes place. When delegates register, they can be asked for their questions. These questions are then useful, both as a guide to the audience's expectations and as a resource to utilise in Q&A sections.

The exact formats in which Q&A can be handled differ depending on the platform or application being used for the presentation.

9.3.3   Third Technique: Gamification

One technique that virtually invariably increases engagement is the introduction of a competitive, gaming element. The best form that gamification should take is related to how big the audience is [1].

9.3.3.1   Gamification for Big Audiences (at Least 150 Attendees)

- Use the generation of a tag cloud or word cloud to break the ice. Set an amusing question and then use software to generate the cloud image. There are several applications which have this functionality. You might ask something provocative, such as "When did you last stay up all night reading something? What was it?"
- Set up a quiz in MCQ format. Alternatively, you might invite certain members of the audience to participate after turning on video and unmuting their microphones. One way to increase the engagement still further is to let the audience choose the category of quiz question. An example of categories for a corporate event might be: "Today's Topic", "History of the Company" or "Little Known Facts".
- Have a competition that runs throughout the event or presentation. This is an especially effective technique when the presentation aims to deliver specific information. You might award points based on answers to specific questions as the presentation unfolds. Attendees have fun watching the leaderboard.
- To increase engagement and a sense of enjoyment generally in an event, you might run polls that are to be answered during the break, with fun questions such as: "Which is better—*The Big Bang Theory* or *Third Rock from the Sun?*" or "Fruit or Cake?" [1].

9.3.3.2   Gamification for Events of No More Than Medium Size (i.e. One Hundred Attendees or Fewer)

- Who said what? You ask the attendees to give a quote on various topics without telling others what they said, then the audience members have to try to match the quote and the person saying it.
- Treasure hunt for use during the midday recess. Set an online challenge that attendees can take part in to find the treasure online. You give them clues and

they can see if they find the treasure. Social media may be used to facilitate the hunt. The suggested answers can be posted online, e.g. on Padlet.

- Pet beauty contest. Ask your audience to submit their favourite photo of their pet so that others can see who has the cutest furry friend.
- Find ten things you have in common. After dividing the whole group up into smaller groups, you can set each group the task of finding ten things they have in common. This is a good way for people who do not normally interact much (or even at all) to learn about others and appreciate how much they have in common. The groups can be sent to individual virtual meeting room or they may converse with each other via chat functionality [1].

9.3.4 Fourth Technique: Encourage Attendees to Network

Networking tends to happen somewhat spontaneously in face-to-face events, but for the same to occur in a virtual environment, there needs to be some specific input from the event organisers or presenters.

Networking can be encouraged in various ways. There are virtual common rooms or lounges available on some platforms or forums, where attendees at an event can begin conversations and start to get to know the other attendees.

You can also assign attendees to breakout rooms and ask everybody in that room to discuss a particular issue. If the groups are not too large, these individuals may turn on their microphones and cameras and talk to each other. A spokesperson can then report on what the group discussed when the whole group returns to the main hall.

One way of planning effectively to allow networking to occur easily at a virtual event is to consider what elements of an F2F event most contribute to the opportunity to network. If you are working with a virtual event facilitator, arrange to reproduce the same opportunities virtually [1].

9.4 Interacting with an Audience Online

Keeping an audience focused on your presentation when the event is online calls for a unique approach. The approaches which are often the most attention-grabbing in an F2F presentation, based on a high energy delivery, may not be as effective when transferred to the online environment. For virtual presentations, the key factor is audience engagement.

The delivery style adopted for virtual presentations needs to fit the presentation medium and the applications you plan to use. Therefore, some changes from F2F will be needed. One key factor to consider is which application is the most appropriate for the presentation you have in mind.

The following tips are all ways to encourage the online audience to pay attention to you, rather than getting distracted onto other tasks, such as checking social media updates or e-mail [2].

9.4.1   Make Yourself More Visible

It is a frequent complaint by online presenters that they cannot observe the audience's reactions. However, it is perhaps a more serious issue that the audience may not be able to see the presenter properly. After all, humans have evolved to pay particular attention to the face during communication.

The work of Robert L. Fantz, dating from 1963, was seminal in understanding the human fascination with faces. This research [3] indicated that babies have a clear preference for the human face over other objects. A further fact to consider is that 90% of communicative content stems from non-verbal elements, namely body language and facial expression. Thus, there is a vital need for the audience to see the presenter's face for maximally effective communication to occur [2].

The most straightforward way to show your face online is by switching on the webcam. Paradoxically, however, many people presenting in a business context actually choose to keep the camera switched off. Indeed, the author has even observed many cases where sales representatives or others have taped over the webcam in order to prevent accidental exposure online. This indicates they are not utilising the potential benefits of increased visibility.

Of course, there are some people who are very reticent about appearing on camera. However, in such cases, at the very least presenters should display a slide showing a picture of themselves and a list of their credentials. This can be put up at the beginning and end of the presentation, as well as when answering questions. The aim is to give yourself human presence, not appear as a disembodied voice, and thus make yourself more engaging.

9.4.2   Use Your Voice to Its Best Advantage

When you are physically present in a place, you need to do more work with your voice. If you adopt a monotonous delivery style, tend to mumble or are indistinct, all of these negative characteristics will be amplified online. Since the voice has such a key role to play in delivery, it is vital to pay close attention to the way you use it.

To begin the process of improving voice delivery, first make a recording of yourself presenting, then examine it critically. There are many online resources offering advice on the best way to improve the quality of your voice. As a minimum, warm-up exercises should be undertaken before presenting. The voice deserves careful treatment and attention from presenters due to its central role in communication.

9.4.3   Be Willing to Allow Pauses

Audiences attending virtual presentations have a certain degree of invisibility and the tendency is to act rather passively. Some presenters respond by speaking much more than they would usually, in an attempt to prevent an uncomfortable silence.

However, this tends to exacerbate the passive tendency of the audience and should be avoided. Learn instead to be comfortable with pauses.

Pauses are, in fact, a very useful way of letting the audience digest the message, ask about any issues they have in understanding or comment. Furthermore, the pause can also be deployed to increase the level of anticipation before delivering a key point, whilst pausing after a key piece of information allows for it to sink in [2].

9.4.4   Begin Punctually

People tend to log on to online presentations in a rather unpunctual manner, often due to problems with connections and entering the correct meeting and logging on details. This then raises the question of whether presenters should wait for late arrivals or begin straightaway.

One way to resolve this dilemma is by starting twice. The first time you start is used to increase audience engagement, but without entering into the key messages of the presentation. This might be termed a "soft beginning".

A soft beginning might involve asking the attendees for an interesting survey question. The question should be clearly relevant and engaging but missing the response should not prevent tardy arrivals from understanding the key messages in the main presentation.

There then follows the second beginning, once everyone has arrived, which is when the presentation proper starts. Whilst staggering the beginning in this way may demand extra effort, it is a good way to ensure the entire audience has a reason to be engaged.

9.4.5   Include Interactive Elements

For engagement to be ongoing throughout the presentation, there should be built-in interactivity. Interaction needs to be carefully planned, rather than left up to chance. Audiences have very short attention spans on average and thus interactivity needs to be frequent to allow them to keep refocusing on the main topic.

A suitable time interval between opportunities to interact should be around once each 4 or 5 min, which is close to the usual attention span. The interaction can consist of various activities, such as asking the audience a question, setting up a survey or using the whiteboard.

Regardless of which type of interactive activity you intend to use, it is important to plan in advance, so that it fits comfortably into the presenting schedule and does not get overlooked under the pressure of presenting [2].

9.4.6   Use Visuals to Strengthen Key Messages

When presentations are delivered F2F, the number of slides required is generally less, since you can more easily observe the audience reactions and decide how well they seem to have understood the message. This kind of feedback is far less online.

The points in a presentation where a recap or a check on understanding should occur are frequently omitted if online presenters mistakenly assume that a silent audience has perfectly understood the message.

To avoid making this mistake and thus leaving your audience behind, at the end of each section be sure to include a slide that reiterates the key points and offers the audience the chance to ask clarifying questions [2].

9.4.7   Paint a Picture with Words

When presenting online, as we previously noted, the words you use are even more vital than in an F2F event. Try to paint a mental picture with the words at your disposal.

Language that evokes a sensory or sensual response is particularly effective in descriptions. Try saying, "it has the colour of a warm summer evening" rather than "it is orange". It is also better to be more precise. Instead of saying, "this is a big machine", say something like, "this computer is the size of three full-size filing cabinets".

Relate your own experiences for extra engagement and make analogies using the audience's terms of reference. It is helpful to listen to good quality podcasts and pick up those features of language use which make the presenter seem engaging and interesting [2].

9.4.8   Keep the Slides Simple

Many people avoid watching the free movie on an international flight because it is difficult to see properly on the back-of-seat screen and demands too much concentration. A similar difficulty often affects audiences at virtual presentations.

The presenter at a virtual presentation has no control over what size device audience members may use to view the presentation. Likewise, not all attendees will have a high-speed connection. You need to assume the slides will be seen on a small screen, where there is a risk that graphics will appear very jumbled. An additional consideration is that an animation may be too laggy or fragmented to be properly understood when broadcast across the internet.

Aim for straightforward, elegant simplicity in laying out the graphic appearance of slides. By not introducing complex animations into slide transitions, you avoid the risk that some attendees will be put off by a disappointing performance [2].

9.4.9 Utilise Movement Carefully

The parts of the brain that can detect movement are amongst the oldest in evolutionary terms. This means that human beings have a well-developed capacity to perceive movement and are naturally drawn towards it. This tendency to fixate on moving objects can be both an advantage and disadvantage for online presenters.

The benefits of movement fascination can be harnessed by having clear transitions between slides and directing the audience's focus using a virtual pointer. However, the disadvantages of this tendency become all too obvious if the video becomes jerky or the mouse is moving erratically across the screen. Be careful to use only those movements which truly add to the presentation and avoid any extraneous movement [2].

9.4.10 Be Punctual in Concluding Your Presentation

Being punctual is an important characteristic that any presenter needs, whether presenting F2F or online. However, a punctual finish is especially important online, as there is a much greater risk of audience members quitting the event before you finish. Be clear about the time-frame and stick to it. Ensure you conclude the presentation within the allotted time and if there are more questions than time permits, arrange to answer them on a separate occasion, or perhaps by e-mail.

Ensuring audience engagement at a virtual presentation is by no means easy to achieve. However, if the presenter appreciates where things are likely to go wrong and plans for such a contingency, the chances of keeping your audience listening attentively throughout are greatly improved [2].

References

1. 4 tools to engage your online audience. Meeting Tomorrow. https://meetingtomorrow.com/blog/engaging-your-audience-online-events/. Accessed 4 Oct 2021.
2. 10 ways to keep your audience engaged during an online presentation. https://visme.co/blog/engage-audience-online-presentation/. Accessed 4 Oct 2021.
3. Geddes L. The big baby experiment. https://www.scientificamerican.com/article/the-big-baby-experiment/. Accessed 4 Oct 2021.

10.1 Introduction

In theory, presentations can range in quality from extremely successful to extremely poor. In practice, however, even those presentations that are of mediocre quality (a good topic, but uninspiring delivery) tend to be remembered as extremely poor. The main reason for a presentation to fail is that it simply bores the audience. Boring presentations harm the reputation of the presenter and make the audience feel tired, demotivated and desperate for the torture to end.

To be able to deliver a highly successful presentation takes practice and meticulous planning of the content. Yet, what gets an audience to sit up and listen with rapt attention is often the way presenters speak and the body language they employ [1].

10.2 How to Maintain Your Audience's Focus and Interest

Maintaining focus and interest from an audience is a more complex task than getting it in the first place. Presentations that are void of interactivity are a highly inefficient method of getting a message across to an audience. They put extreme demands on the audience in terms of remaining silent and focused for lengthy stretches of time. Rather than expecting your audience to do all the work, there are seven ways in which you can naturally increase their focus and interest [2], as we will see in the following sections.

10.2.1 Pick a Topic That Your Audience Already Wants to Know About

Although it seems like a somewhat elementary error to make, it is in fact surprisingly common to find presenters confusing what they themselves find interesting

C. C. Cingi et al., *Improving Online Presentations*,
https://doi.org/10.1007/978-3-031-28328-4_10

with what audience members want to know. An example of making this mistake might be the following. Suppose a clinical biochemist is asked to speak to medical students about laboratory investigations. The students will most likely be focused on the clinical value of the tests, in other words, how they can use them effectively in patients. If the biochemist instead talks about the minutiae of laboratory analytical technique (which is her main interest), the talk is likely to fall flat and leave the audience unsatisfied.

It is also important not to decide to change the subject of the presentation after the audience have already signed up for it. Suppose a hundred people sign up for a session billed as an "Introduction to Fintech (financial technology)". They are expecting an introduction into the field and an explanation of why technology is acting as a disruptor in financial markets. The presenter may be an expert in the field but has developed instead an interest in security of online banking. However expertly the presentation is delivered, the chances of the audience being satisfied with the switched topic are slim. When this recently occurred, only 5 of the audience members expressed satisfaction with the talk when a feedback survey was given.

10.2.2 Give People Reasons for Listening

Prior to giving a presentation, it may be a good idea to get your audience to complete an online survey asking them for their views on the importance of the topic you are due to present. If the answers indicate that there are individuals who are not yet convinced why the topic is important, it will be well worth spending the first part of the presentation outlining persuasive reasons for learning about the topic. For example, a presenter talking about communication skills in a business environment might give a real life example of when communication skills had helped to close a deal or how developing these skills has led to previous attendees getting promoted. Once there is a reason to listen, the audience will be more focused on what you have to say.

Thus, where you may have an audience without a prior interest in a topic, you may need to spend time winning them around to be interested first. This may be a difficult task if the topic appears highly technical or not obviously related to the audience's current preoccupations. For example, it may be difficult to get some audiences interested in password security. However, if the presenter explains the personal consequences of password theft, the topic may take on a new relevance. A colleague of the author relates how there was a lax approach to password security in her department. Several members of staff shared a password to access a particular database. When an incident occurred related to the database, the employee to whom the password was originally assigned was called on to explain why he had accessed data inappropriately. When unable to do so, his employment was terminated. After telling this story, the audience shared a few guilty looks and then listened attentively throughout the presentation that followed.

Of course, the corollary to this argument is that if the presenter cannot find a reason why the audience should be interested, it is better not to deliver the presentation at all [2].

10.2.3 Avoid Both Over-Simplification and Over-Complication

In psychology, there is a concept termed "flow", investigated by Csikszentmihalyi [3], which refers to a psychological state where a person is pleasantly and totally absorbed in the activity he or she is undertaking. When a person experiences this psychological state, focus is easily maintained and the sense of time passing is lost. Presentations that are perceived as "fascinating" or "compelling" are ones where the audience has entered a flow state. Indeed, it can be said that all presentations ultimately share the ideal objective of putting the audience members into a state of flow [4].

The flow state depends on many different factors; however, a key consideration is that the level of concentration and mental effort required should be neither too little nor too great. Attending to a presentation calls for mental exertion in order to understand and follow the messages given. Therefore, this degree of exertion should be optimal for the type of audience who will attend. Calibrating the level of the presentation to achieve this target means the presenter needs to know the previous level of knowledge the audience already has about a topic and how confident they are in expanding that knowledge.

A presenter who simply reads off a list of bullet points from a slide is giving the audience so little mental stimulation that they will easily get bored.

Conversely, if a presenter displays a highly complex infographic and immediately begins discussing the minutiae without giving an initial overview, the cognitive effort required to understand the presentation is liable to be too great for the audience. They stop listening. The psychologist, Daniel T. Willingham, describes an experiment in which he took a group of students, told them to pay attention and then gave them rapid cognitive overload. Virtually all the students lost their focus within 15 s [5]. This study identified mismatch of the effort required to understand and the students' ability to do so as a key reason for disliking learning a topic.

Accordingly, you should see your presentation in terms of how much effort the audience will need to exert to understand each section. Aim for material that requires some effort but is not overwhelming [2].

10.2.4 Alterations Attract Attention

It is well-established in psychology that alterations or changes are things the human mind focuses on [5]. When a motorcycle engine starts loudly outside a lecture hall, the students tend to be distracted by it. However, unless it is very loud, after a whilst the students tend to filter out the noise. It only then becomes apparent again when the noise changes again, when the motorcycle drives away.

This focus on alteration can be used to direct an audience's attention. It is convenient to divide alterations up into macro- and micro-alterations [2].

10.2.4.1   Macro-alterations

Examples include:

1. Altering the presentation medium, such as moving from a projected presentation to a whiteboard or vice versa.
2. Getting the presentation attendees to stand up and move around the room, perhaps to participate in an activity.
3. Altering where you stand to present, such as moving across to the other side of the room.
4. Altering between passive listening and some other type of activity, such as doing some pair work with another attendee.
5. Switching between presenters.
6. Moving to a different topic.

10.2.4.2   Micro-alterations

Micro-alterations also help to refocus audience attention. The following are some examples of how to create a micro-alteration.

1. Mark the divisions between subtopics clearly, by saying something such as: "That is the issue with X. Let's now move onto a different topic". Emphasising movement (a type of alteration) prompts the listener to sit up and pay attention to the new material.
2. Let the audience watch a brief video clip.
3. Pause before, and after, making a particularly important point.
4. Alter the style of delivery depending on what type of material you are presenting. If you are discussing data or other facts, speak in a more serious tone than you would use to relate an anecdote, which you may present in a more conversational tone.

In general, the advice is to have a macro-alteration occur every 10 min or even more frequently, whilst micro-alterations can occur virtually continuously.

10.2.5 Adopt a Storytelling Style

The tremendously powerful technique of storytelling is something any highly skilled presenter will be familiar with. It appears that humans have evolved naturally to be interested in hearing stories. Every time a presenter mentions a story is about to come, there is an up-tick in the audience focus and interest. Naturally, using stories works best if they have a clear relevance to the topic of the presentation. Stories are more effective if they are spread throughout a presentation, rather than only in one or two sections.

It is also possible to structure the entire presentation in the form of stories or a main story. There are various ways to do this, which are discussed elsewhere [2].

10.2.6 Insert Breaks Frequently

Ensure that breaks are inserted frequently in any series of presentations, but be prepared also to offer a micro-break, lasting for at most a couple of minutes, if the audience appear to be getting fatigued. Getting people to stand up for a few moments works well to dispel a tendency to sleepiness [2].

10.2.7 Keep Presentations Brief

Keeping a presentation relatively brief is the best way to ensure that the audience do not lose their focus before the end.

10.3   Extra Ways to Keep the Audience Focused

The following are all techniques presenters can use to get the audience to focus on the presentation [1]:

10.3.1 Begin with a Surprise

It is best not to begin presenting in an undistinguished, completely conventional way. Assuming you have a new or surprising angle on your topic, you can drop enticing hints about what lies in store. Imagine that you have a presentation about the future of your industry. Start by painting a provocative picture of how that future may look. If you can generate interest from the very beginning of the presentation and give an enticing glimpse of what is to come, your audience will start to hang on your every word. Just as you can start with an imaginative picture, so you can show some shocking statistic or some highly revealing piece of information.

10.3.2 Narrate a Tale

Human beings have a natural preference for hearing tales. The storytelling ability appears to be an evolutionary adaptation to enable cultures to pass on their experience. This ability means that audiences can follow and understand stories more readily than facts, figures and arguments. Try to cast as much of the information you have to provide in story-form as possible. Tie the tale together with actual or imagined experiences. Let metaphor work for you to show the connections between ideas. The greater the degree of storytelling within a presentation, the higher the level of audience engagement.

10.3.3 Do Not Restrict Yourself to a Script

Of course, before delivering a presentation, it is always good practice to be well-prepared and to have practised delivery several times. However, at the actual presentation, be prepared to range further than the script. The aim of practising delivery is to be familiar enough with the material that you can adapt the presentation and talk in a more spontaneous fashion. Audiences appreciate the difference between when you speak spontaneously and when you are simply well-rehearsed.

10.3.4 Let Your Voice Convey Emotions

If your material inspires no emotions in you at all, it might be prudent to pass the job onto someone else. You should let the audience hear the emotion in your voice at different stages of the presentation. If you are telling the audience a shocking reality, you should sound shocked. If you say that you are excited by a solution, sound excited! Avoid a bland tone, which makes the material sound flat and irrelevant. Your emotions guide the audience how they should feel about what you are saying. Only robots lack emotion.

10.3.5 Using Contrasting Volume Levels in Your Voice

A presentation delivered in a constant tone is exactly that, monotonous. Likewise, volume levels should fluctuate to maintain variety. The key points and salient facts can be highlighted by volume contrasts in delivery. When the material is more routine, you need not speak particularly loudly, but you can build to a climax as you reveal the key points you want the audience to grasp.

10.3.6 Vary the Pace of Delivery

In the same way that emotional tone and volume should vary somewhat, so should the pace of delivery. Speak at one comfortable pace for background information or when summarising a section but speak more slowly and deliberately when you have a vital message to deliver. Be prepared to pause silently after slowing down. Do, however, be careful that the changes in pace do not themselves become tediously repetitive.

10.3.7 Address Particular Members of the Audience

If you want to address specific people, you will need to exercise a certain amount of flexibility, since those particular individuals may not be present, and their willingness to be involved may vary. Nonetheless, getting some audience members to take part increases the overall level of engagement. The individuals may be invited to come up to the front, turn on their cameras (if online) or be less actively involved. In the latter case, you might simply refer to that person by name.

10.3.8 Inject Some Humour

Whatever the topic, an injection of humour typically helps. Humour is an element that makes the audience happy and makes them want to focus on what you are saying. Whilst presenters should be aware of the danger of crossing the boundary of acceptability with certain jokes, a gentle approach to humour is usually a great way for a presenter to become more appealing to an audience.

10.3.9 Do Not Bombard the Audience with Facts and Figures

Unless absolutely essential, many facts and figures can be confined to background slides, allowing interested members of the audience to follow them up later. A presentation should not be just a form of spoken textbook. An engaging presentation gives the audience insights and access to new ideas.

10.3.10 Avoid Simply Reading

A presentation where the presenter just reads off the same words written on the slides is bound to be a disastrous failure. Not only is it extremely tedious, it also makes the audience feel the presenter does not trust them to be able to read for themselves. Needless to say, this technique should never be used. Talk around the slides, using different words.

There is no reason for a presentation to be dull unless a presenter decides to make it so. By following the advice in this book, including this chapter, your presentations should always be engaging, illuminating and enjoyable to watch [1].

References

1. 10 presentation tricks to keep your audience awake. https://www.inc.com/jayson-demers/10-presentation-tricks-to-keep-your-audience-awake.html. Accessed 4 Oct 2021.
2. Mitchell O. 7 ways to keep audience attention during your presentation. https://speakingabout-presenting.com/content/7-ways-audience-attention-presentation/. Accessed 4 Oct 2021.

3. https://en.wikipedia.org/wiki/Mihaly_Csikszentmihalyi. Accessed 4 Oct 2021.
4. When giving presentations, the only rule that matters is the rule of attention. 2 Nov 2009. https://finiteattentionspan.wordpress.com/2009/11/02/the-only-rule-about-giving-presentations-that-matters-is-the-rule-of-attention/. Accessed 4 Oct 2021.
5. Willingham DT. Why don't students like school?: A cognitive scientist answers questions about how the mind works and what it means for the classroom. 2nd ed. Hoboken: Jossey Bass; 2021. ISBN-13: 978-0470279304. https://www.amazon.com/Why-Dont-Students-Like-School/dp/0470279303%3FSubscriptionId%3DAKIAI4VN2TG2UUWEVTBQ%26tag%3Dwwwspeakingab-20%26linkCode%3Dxm2%26camp%3D2025%26creative%3D165953%26creativeASIN%3D0470279303. Accessed 4 Oct 2021.

Achieving Maximum Effectiveness in Presenting

11

11.1 Presenting Effectively

The visual elements of a presentation make a greater impact on audiences than the verbal elements, as effective presenters are aware. This greater impact is due to the fact that humans have more highly evolved vision than other senses.

Furthermore, the key role played in communication by non-verbal signals generally has been amply demonstrated through academic research. A study, which looked at the effects of communicating single words, ascertained that the expression on the speaker's face carried 55% of the message, the tone of voice 38% and the word itself only 7%. This research was carried out by Albert Mehrabian in the Psychology Faculty of UCLA. Whilst one limitation of this finding is that only single words were used and the setting was a research laboratory, one conclusion is clear: it is misplaced effort to concentrate on the choice of words used but neglect the manner in which those words will be delivered.

Thus, this chapter outlines a more rational strategy for how to ensure your presentation achieves the greatest possible impact. The strategy outlined consists of achieving three goals, which together lead to presentation success.

The first goal, which is also the most essential, is to connect on an emotional level with the audience. Unless this connection exists, the message will be less effectively delivered. The second goal is to achieve a highly energetic performance, which will capture the attention of the audience and ensure it remains focused on the presenter throughout delivery. The final goal is to make sure the content supplies a clearly visible benefit for the audience members.

It is common for presentations to fail to achieve these goals. Where the goals are achieved, however, presenters enjoy a significantly greater degree of success than is otherwise possible [1].

C. C. Cingi et al., *Improving Online Presentations*,
https://doi.org/10.1007/978-3-031-28328-4_11

11.1.1 Connecting Emotionally with Audiences

Whether or not the audience members are consciously aware of doing so, they will have formed an initial impression of a presenter in a matter of seconds. This impression may be positive or negative. Indeed, despite many people insisting they do not act on their first impressions, which are apt to be misinformed, this appears to be a normal human psychological response. The effective delivery of a message in a presentation depends on this initial audience "chemistry". For the audience to accept a message, the presenter should appear to be someone the audience may like and trust.

There is a straightforward way for presenters to increase their likeability, which is to demonstrate warmth towards the audience. Presenters should look around the audience before starting the presentation, establishing eye contact and exchanging a few smiles. This warmth tends to be reciprocated. Audiences trust likeable presenters more. Being enthusiastic also conveys likeability.

At all stages in delivering a presentation, try to maintain eye contact with the listeners. Failing to keep eye contact conveys a very negative impression, such as that you have no wish to present, do not genuinely believe in the message you are giving or possibly that you cannot be trusted. Conversely, a speech delivered with genuine positive emotion conveys the idea of sincerity. If the audience observes your belief, they will also tend to accept the message. Ensure that you can deliver your presentation without needing to look down at cue cards, by practising well. Reliance on cue cards tends to prevent eye contact with the audience and constrains your emotional responses to the message.

Above all, try to establish common ground with the audience. Do not appear lofty or unreachable. Act with some humility. Share experiences that show you are only human, too, and demonstrate commitment to values that the audience also share. Tell stories, since stories appeal to all types of people.

It is important for the audience to perceive the presenter as knowledgeable about the topic. It is better to let another individual introduce you and warmly endorse your credentials as a presenter than for you to list your own credentials.

Likeability depends to an extent on similarity. Establish as much common ground with the audience as you can, but do not become fake by stretching this too far. Refer to people or resources that the audience are already familiar with and respect. Show that you share some of the audience's emotions. In terms of dress, it is best to be slightly smarter in appearance than most of the members of the audience.

On occasions where a presentation involves conveying bad news to an audience, make it clear that you empathise with your audience's likely reaction. Be specific about details, such as times and individuals involved, so that the audience realise you know the full picture. Where an opposing argument exists for what you are advocating, it is wise to show that you are familiar with it, demonstrate fairness about the strengths of the opposing argument and ultimately be able to justify why your own view is superior. Ignoring an opposing view may suggest to an audience that you cannot answer the objection. Where an apology is required, it should be delivered in a frank and straightforward way. Audiences do not like presenters who speak obliquely and use euphemisms all the time. Explain that you can take questions or comments at the end of your presentation and ensure there is adequate time to do so.

When you present after other speakers, it is best to attend early, listen carefully to their presentations and refer to them when it is your time to present. By sitting in the audience first, you send a message of solidarity with the audience. If a presenter can arrive early at an event and introduce herself to some members of the audience before the presentations begin, rapport and connection will be easier to establish when the time arrives for her to deliver her own presentation [1].

11.1.2 Deliver an Energetic Presentation

Introduce a story full of drama at the very start of the presentation, if you want to begin energetically and get the audience enthused from the very beginning. If you want the audience to feel excitement about the material you are presenting, they need to feel the presenter's excitement first.

Enter the room of the presentation with your shoulders back, head up, and convey confidence in your posture and movement. Look around at the audience before beginning to speak. Use your body language to emphasise particular points in the presentation. You can gesticulate with your arms and head. Make sure your face expresses the appropriate emotions. Use a range of volume in speaking and vary the pace, remembering to pause when you really want to emphasise a point. Speak using short sentences, avoid passive sentences (the active is much easier to comprehend) and use rhetorical techniques, like the use of onomatopoeia (words with a sound that reflects their meaning, like "crash", "tinkle" or "splash"). Speak plainly, without constantly qualifying what you say. Make use of a variable distance between yourself and the audience. Indeed, some presenters actually like to get in amongst the audience, to ask for an opinion, for example. Be sure that you sleep well before a presentation, so that you can throw yourself into it with boundless energy.

Keep a close eye on how the audience are reacting. If they seem to be getting tired, change what you are doing. Make use of a sudden change of pace, adjust the speaking volume, show an unexpected prop, pose a challenge to your audience or get them to interact. All these techniques maintain the energy of the presentation.

Do remember, however, that presentations should not be too long. The more senior the audience you face, the less willing they become to listen to a lengthy presentation. Audiences are always happy when a presentation lasts a shorter time than the full time slot and if the presentation style has been energetic throughout [1].

11.1.3 Make It Clear What the Audience Gain by Listening

When a presentation is educational or supplies information, presenters should emphasise how relevant and applicable the information is, rather than attempting to give comprehensive details. To persuade an audience to make a change in their behaviour, you need to show them that the change will be beneficial for them as individuals. Convincing an audience involves both a rational and an emotional appeal. You need to provide convincing evidence to show that your argument is rational, and emotional appeal by emphasising how the solution you offer will make life easier or more enjoyable in some way.

Even if it may seem extremely self-evident to the presenter what the benefits are, it would be wrong to assume the audience will feel the same. You need to use every technique to persuade them. Show the relevance of the key messages by showing how they apply in practice. Use analogy when explaining. Make the message easier to remember by use of acronyms (abbreviations that spell out a word), alliteration (repetition of the same sound) and rhyming phrases: MIME—Make It Memorable for Everyone, Splendid Splashing Sparkling Spa Water, Give your customers the very best, Then they'll forget all the rest.

Given how great a role visual learning plays in most people, you should make extensive use of visuals when presenting. However, do not let the visuals become so spectacular that the audience attention shifts away from you onto the visuals. A few, straightforward but attractive visuals are usually sufficient. After all, you want the audience to listen to your message rather than feel they are watching a demonstration of PowerPoint's latest features. Concentrate on making a connection with your audience before you roll out the big (visual) guns [1].

11.2   Advice on How to Use PowerPoint Effectively

Make use of the master slide design feature so that the entire slide set has a consistent look. Individual slides can deviate in their content and layout, such as single or double column text, bullet-point lists, accompanying images, etc. However, the colour scheme, any background artwork and fonts should be consistent throughout the presentation.

Keep down the word count on each slide and simplify wherever possible. Just highlight the key points and put the minimum information required to get the correct message across.

Avoid complex punctuation and avoid the use of ALL UPPER CASE. This comes across as shouting. Leaving some blank areas on a slide makes it much easier to read.

The text must stand out clearly from the background. Choose a colour scheme that will be easily legible when projected (i.e. high contrast). Text stands out better if it is light on dark than the other way around. Background images or artwork should not be distracting.

Keep the transitions between slides simple and easy to follow. Some of the transition effects, such as fly-ins, have an initial appeal but may actually detract from the presentation overall by seeming too "gimmicky". This, in turn, may reduce the level of trust the audience has in the presenter.

When using images, ensure they are of high quality and serve to strengthen the message of your presentation. It is important to check how the images will appear when they appear on a projector screen or on a mobile device.

A "build slide" is one where you keep adding lines of text to a slide as you present. Whilst this may be useful, avoid the situation where text keeps appearing from different directions. The text should enter from the left of the screen, or from above. Build slides tend to slow down a presentation and therefore should be employed sparingly.

Avoid an excessive number of slides. If your presentation involves near-constant switching from one slide to another, your audience will quickly tire. In general, a rate of one slide each minute works well.

You should be able to present without needing always to follow the same order. The software allows you to skip ahead or go back to any slide in the presentation without needing to flick through all the intervening slides.

It is vital to know how to navigate through a slide set easily, for the frequent occasions when an audience member is interested in viewing a particular slide a second time.

When you practise before delivering the presentation, it is a good idea to check how well the slides project with the equipment you will be using on the day of the actual presentation. Check if the text on slides is legible for audience members situated right at the back. The text should be of sufficient size to ensure legibility, but not so large that it seems to be shouting at the audience.

Prepare a backup plan in case PowerPoint or the projector is not working properly. It is wise to bring handouts and even overhead projector transparencies. However, remember that any animated effects will be lost when you change medium, so be prepared to explain without the animation.

Be prepared to do a dress rehearsal for your presentation with someone who has not seen it previously. Solicit that person's views on the colour scheme, the content, any visuals and use of special effects.

Never just read from the slides. The audience can read the slides for themselves.

Face the audience, not the screen. A common mistake some presenters make is to look in the direction of the screen when they should be addressing the audience in front of them.

Avoid making excuses for material that the audience will struggle to understand. If the material is too complex, it is better to omit it from the presentation [2].

11.3 How to Avoid PowerPoint Disasters

PowerPoint is the current market leader for preparing slides to be used in commercial and other presentations. The software makes it a straightforward task to create a set of slides that are visually appealing and can be easily updated as required. Despite this ease of use and its many advantages, PowerPoint can just as easily help to produce a presenting disaster as a presenting success. The most important principal is to use PowerPoint to showcase your presentation, rather than your presentation to showcase PowerPoint. To achieve the highest level of success, take heed of the following tips.

Transitions between slides and audio features If unwisely used, slide transitions and sound effects may take the audience's attention away from the key message of a slide. Even more disastrous is when a PowerPoint show is run on a system with too low a specification. The show ends up running very slowly and in a distorted way that either makes you laugh or cry with frustration. In fact, for the majority of presentations, these hi-tech gimmicks can be omitted. They may be suitable if you want to create a comical or kitsch presentation, but otherwise are best laid aside. After all, a presentation does not need to resemble a cinematic special effect *tour de force* to be successful! Even relatively simple special effects, such as build slides, need to be used very sparingly. The message is much more vital than any PowerPoint bells and whistles.

Out-of-the-box clip-art The standard clip-art bundled with PowerPoint looks tired and hackneyed. It is best avoided unless you want your presentation to look like a clone of other presentations. Using this clip-art makes your presentation appear unoriginal. So, a better approach is to think how graphics can help to get the message across. Are graphics really necessary? Where the graphics do serve a definite purpose, you can use your own digital or digitised photographs. There are also providers of high quality images online, such as Photodisc (www.photodisc.com) or Hemera's Photo Objects (www.hemera.com). A screenshot may be a valuable graphical aid when talking about software or a web-based resource. If you want to perform a screen capture, two useful applications are Snagit (www.techsmith.com) for Windows or Snapz Pro (www.ambrosiasw.com) for Mac users, which can both be licensed as shareware.

Presentation templates Presentation templates also often appear outdated. When you use a standard template, it restricts how creative you can be. Furthermore, the colour schemes employed are often ill-chosen and any background images tend to distract attention from the rest of the slide. A better idea is to read up on best practice in creating graphics for the web and use the same approach to choose the colour scheme and layout for the slide master. Let the slides be clearly original and place any logo for your organisation on one corner of the slide.

Slides with too much text Slides work well when they summarise a concept in graphical form or supply the overview for a topic. Where they are much less effective is in supplying fine detail. Text should be kept short and in notes form. There should be no complete paragraphs of text, extended quotations or lengthy sentences. At most the length of text should not exceed five lines per slide. Use single words or brief phrases rather than sentences. That way, the audience have a greater chance of reading the slide and comprehending the message. The slides are not the same as either the speaker notes or the presentation outline. They reinforce the message of the presentation.

Remember the audience perspective Many presenters succumb to the temptation to paste data or graphics directly from printed material onto slides. This is virtually never a good idea since printed materials differ from projected slides in several respects. For a start, printed matter is generally intended to be viewed from 20 to 30 cm away, whereas the audience is usually at least 1 or 2 m from the screen. The images reproduced in printed materials are generally too small, contain too much detail and have too much text to work well when projected onto a screen. Most readers can comfortably read a font at 12 points. However, a slide is very hard to read if the font is less than 40 points. Think of the audience's perspective and ensure that any material is in a format that will not induce eye strain.

Spoken vs. written language Presenters should always deliver a presentation interactively, by speaking to an audience, not by reading a pre-prepared speech. The form of language varies considerably between speaking and writing. Whereas written language tends to be complicated, more qualified and more formal, effective spoken language is brief, to-the-point and less concerned with formality. If you read your presentation, it will never sound completely natural.

If you plan to distribute a written handout to your audience, think about the best time to do so. Audiences tend to read the materials you give them, rather than listen to your explanation. Furthermore, if they know everything you plan to say, there is little incentive to remain focused on listening. Keep the audience guessing what is coming next by not supplying handouts until the end of the presentation.

Over-reliance on technology When you deliver a presentation, never assume all your equipment will work exactly as you planned. Devices may need to be updated and networks may fail to recognise your laptop or notebook. Always keep multiple copies of your presentation, perhaps on a USB flash memory and a cloud-based storage solution. If the copy is easily accessible, it can still be adjusted at the last minute to cope with unexpected changes. Even in the era of ubiquitous digital projectors, having overhead projector transparencies as a backup is valuable, at least for the most important slides. If you are very unlucky, there may be a power cut and you will have nothing to show at all. Be prepared for such a contingency by knowing the content of the presentation inside-out and know how to give a spontaneous speech-only presentation. Being able to present without technological backup is a rare ability, but one definitely worth acquiring [2].

11.4   Advice on PowerPoint Settings

Fonts
- Use a consistent font throughout the presentation. Fonts which lack serifs, e.g. *Arial* or *Gill Sans*, project more effectively than fonts with serifs, such as *Times New Roman* or *Palatino*, which are more suited to printed materials.
- The minimum font size on any slide should be 24 points.

- All titles and headings in the presentation should be written in the same font.
- Use a different font for the headlines than for the rest of the text.
- Captions or subheadings should be in bold and a different size from the main body of text.
- Yet another font is needed if sidebars or page numbers are included.
- The maximum number of different fonts that you should use in a presentation is four.
- Every slide should carry a clear title. The title should be in point size 35–45, or a different colour from the rest of the slide.
- The use of larger-sized text indicates material which is more important.
- To achieve a greater impact, vary the text size, colour and effect (such as bold).
- It is best to avoid *italics*, as they are less legible than regular script.
- Keep sentences brief.
- Unless essential, do not use abbreviations or acronyms.
- Punctuate sparingly.
- Each line should contain a maximum 6–8 words.
- For lists consisting of bullet points, there should be no more than 6 words on each line and maximum six lines in total (the "6 × 6 rule").
- Text should be either dark on a light background, or vice versa. It is worth bearing in mind that some individuals find light text on a dark background harder to read than dark on light.
- The only time ALL CAPITALS is appropriate is for titles.
- If you insert a repeating element, such as the slide number, keep its position constant on different slides.
- A good guide to legibility is whether you can read comfortably when standing 2 m away from the projector screen.

Slide Design and Use of Graphics
- Apply a template to the design.
- Be consistent in where you place items, the colour scheme used and the styles adopted.
- Avoid unnecessary content.
- In other words, only include the essential.
- Appropriate content can speak for itself.
- Contrasting or complementary colours are best.
- Keep the total number of slides low so the audience does not give up.
- Slide backgrounds should be unobtrusive and the same in each slide.
- Have few transitions, ideally just one, so it does not become distracting.
- Use a consistent style for bullet points.
- If you have a header, keep any graphics the same on all slides.
- A single large image, or a couple, is preferable to multiple smaller pictures on the slide.
- Just showcase the important images; otherwise. the audience does not know which images they should pay most attention to.
- The image size should be consistent.

- Borders should remain constant.
- Images may be placed in a vertical or horizontal order.
- Text that accompanies graphics should be both concise and precise.
- Avoid a messy or cluttered look. Make use of empty space.
- If you need to use clip-art, it should be a high quality image and clearly relevant to the topic. Only use clip-art if it definitely makes the message clearer.
- Any images employed in a presentation should generally be of the same type, such as all cartoons or photographs.
- Do not place too many images on a single slide.
- Repeating an image may be helpful in reinforcing a point.
- Remember that you can edit a single clip-art image in various ways to give greater variety. For example, the size can be altered, as can the colour. Images can also be reversed or flipped horizontally.
- If you want an image to clearly stand out, make sure it is in a clearly contrasting colour from the rest of the slide.
- Always confirm before the presentation itself that images project satisfactorily on a screen.
- The use of very striking images and animations with sound effects runs the risk of distracting the audience from the main message, so should only be used if genuinely valuable.

Colour
- Use a restricted number of different colours on any one slide.
- Although bright colours generally let small objects and slender lines stand out, the colour may not project effectively.
- A chart should contain a maximum of four different colours.
- Remember that the colour as it appears on a computer screen (or monitor) will be different from when projected. Check the projected colour for acceptability prior to the event.

General Advice on Presenting
- Prepare meticulously.
- Research the topic well.
- Analyse your audience.
- Practise timing.
- Speak in a clear and comfortable way.
- Ensure there are no grammatical or spelling mistakes.
- Avoid reading out a presentation. Practise so that cue cards are sufficient to allow you to speak. There is a difference between the slides and the cue cards. The slides are for the audience, the cue cards are for the presenter.
- Begin with an overview, then move on to the key points, before ending by reiterating the main message.
- It may be better to have a list appear in stages as you present, rather than have the whole list visible from the start. The gradual reveal prevents the audience from simply reading the list and ignoring the presenter.

- If you are using the mouse, a cordless model lets you walk around with it in your hand.
- Any audio (including sound effects) should have stopped playing before you try to speak.
- For complex topics, it may be helpful to print out the slides and let the audience members annotate their copies.
- Do not turn away from the audience. Place the laptop screen in such a way that you can see both it and the audience [2].

References

1. Making an effective presentation. 24 Feb 2010. https://www.forbes.com/2010/02/24/effective-presentation-skills-leadership-careers-rosenthal.html?sh=7ead166430cf. Accessed 4 Oct 2021.
2. Sommerville J. Tips for making effective PowerPoint presentations. https://www.ncsl.org/legislators-staff/legislative-staff/legislative-staff-coordinating-committee/tips-for-making-effective-powerpoint-presentations.aspx. Accessed 24 Oct 2021.

12.1 Tone of Voice

The tone of voice you adopt when presenting conveys an image of what your organisation values and believes and is thus an element of presenting that calls for serious consideration. Everyone knows how a remark spoken in a certain tone of voice can create anger or sadness, and the same effect is created when speaking to clients or other professionals. It is important to avoid alienating others by an inappropriate tone of voice [1].

12.1.1 Your Voice Conveys Your Identity

Hitting the right tone when speaking allows you to market yourself most effectively. When speaking to other business people, an appropriate tone would probably sound sober, business-like and professional. Conversely, addressing a gathering of adolescents may call for a more humorous and playful tone. It is important to keep up a consistent tone of voice and thus create your own brand identity. Ensure it is a tone that appeals to your clients. However, avoid assuming a fake identity in an attempt to be more likeable. If a brand is sober and professional, do not adopt a teasing tone. After all, there are many tones of voice you can adopt and the one chosen should sound genuine and unaffected [1].

12.1.2 Tone of Voice Differentiates You from Others

The passion, calm or anger in your tone of voice all have an effect on how your audience see you. Without a particular tone of voice, everybody sounds the same and no particular voice would ever stand out. Tone of voice conveys the innovative, exciting edge a company can bring to business. It can make you seem warm, experienced,

C. C. Cingi et al., *Improving Online Presentations*, https://doi.org/10.1007/978-3-031-28328-4_12

able to see the funny side and lets you showcase any side of your business persona that you want others to notice. It makes you a unique-sounding individual [1].

12.1.3 Tone of Voice Helps Establish Trustworthiness

As people listen to the tone of voice you are speaking in, they are forming an impression of the personality behind the voice and imaging how the organisation you are representing must be. These judgements bring the audience a sense of being familiar with the organisation and thus they start to increase their trust in you and your organisation.

It is reassuring for clients to encounter consistency of tone in any of the channels they use to approach your organisation. These channels may be telephone, e-mail or any social media. Consistency conveys the impression the organisation has genuine values and clients feel more reassured that their expectations will be met [1].

12.1.4 Tone May Help You Be More Influential and Persuasive

Having established they are trustworthy in the eyes of prospective clients, presenters can rely on this impression to be more influential and persuasive, moving the client to commit to a business relationship. People naturally prefer to transact business with individuals or organisations that appear more likeable and trustworthy.

There is thus a compelling business argument for an organisation to discover its corporate identity and use that to decide on the tone of voice used when communicating. Organisations should first decide on their values and the perception they wish to create, then guarantee these values are reflected in all the touch points. In some organisations, brand guidelines are formulated to reflect this need. Following such guidelines means the organisation can craft a consistent perception in the minds of both its own employees and clients and move on from being one company amongst many to a company with a definite brand identity [1].

12.1.5 Use of the Voice When Presenting

The voice is a vital tool for getting your message delivered effectively. The way the voice is used makes all the difference between words that ring out brightly and those that disappear into the shadows [2].

12.1.5.1   Projecting and Articulating

The volume of the voice needs to be sufficiently loud and clear for the audience to catch each word and understand the meaning. The correct level is achieved when everyone, whether in the front row or at the back, can hear without struggling to do so. A well-projected delivery also conveys you have a compelling personality.

A powerful voice makes you seem confident. A voice that is overly soft, indistinct or trails off conveys to the audience that you feel uncertain or hesitant. This apparent lack of conviction then undermines the message you want to deliver. If presenters feel certain words or phrases lack real significance, they should jettison those parts of the presentation. It is far better to deliver what remains with genuine confidence.

Making a message more audible gives your audience an easier time and makes you a more effective communicator. Anything that prevents a clear delivery will detract from the value of your presentation.

If there is a microphone present, it certainly helps with increasing the volume, but increased volume can never compensate for a weak delivery that lacks personal warmth [2].

12.1.5.2 Pace

It is easy for a person reading an article to re-read any sections where the meaning was not immediately obvious. However, this is not possible when listening to a live presentation. The presenter needs instead to maintain a pace that gives sufficient time to the audience to comprehend the key messages. This kind of pace also permits presenters to consider carefully the content of their words and to ensure that the way they are presenting is giving the correct message [2].

12.1.5.3 Variety

Variation in voice levels adds a distinctive vocal flavour to a presentation. Whilst presenting, there should be variations in tone of voice, pace and how loud the speech is.

Listening to a voice that lacks this variety causes audiences to lose their concentration and cease paying attention. It is surely highly significant that the adjective describing this style of speech, monotonous, is synonymous with "tedious" or "boring".

Presenters who are comfortable with their topic and enthusiastic about the content of the presentation tend to vary their speech in this way spontaneously. These variations cast a light on how the presenter sees the material (exciting, alarming, etc.) and this guides the listeners' appreciation of the content. Not only is the material easier to comprehend, it also becomes more interesting [2].

12.1.5.4 Inflection

One frequently encountered problem in vocal delivery involves the pitch levels at different points in the sentence, i.e. intonation. In English, a rising pitch at the end of a sentence converts a statement into a question. Thus, even a simple word, like "danger" can be made into "danger?" by raising the pitch at the end. Normal statements do not have this feature. Consider the same word used as a warning: "danger!".

It is characteristic of some speakers that they overuse the rising tone, applying it even to statements where there should be no rise in pitch. This produces the impression that the speaker lacks confidence in what he or she is saying and needs confirmation from the listener.

Furthermore, rising intonation may imply that the speaker has incompletely expressed his or her idea and wants to continue. This may make the audience falsely conclude that the next statement is part of the same sentence, which may lead to confusion [2]. Compare the following:

1. "No, I don't. Like John, I prefer Georgia" with
2. "No I don't like John. I prefer Georgia".

Inappropriate use of a rising tone when saying sentence (1) may make the listeners perceive (2). John just became your enemy!

Thus, incorrect application of rising tone can be both confusing and make speakers sound unsure of themselves.

12.1.5.5 Silences

Using silence is a powerful technique.

Silence can be used at various points to focus your listeners' attention. A silence before you begin speaking commands attention, as does a pause after a key statement. It adds emphasis. More than that, judicious use of silences sends a message that presenters are confident enough in what they are saying to let the audience dwell for a moment on the significance of their remarks. Consider the difference between a dignified silence and someone speaking so fast that he almost forgets to draw his own breath.

However, presenters frequently feel uncomfortable with silence and may respond by filling in the gaps with "umm"s and "agh"s. This tendency should definitely be avoided as it quickly becomes tedious for an audience and comes across as lack of confidence from the speaker.

Instead of filling in the gaps like this, when you need to think what to say next, pause briefly and then continue as the thoughts come into your mind. A presenter usually perceives a gap to think in a presentation as far longer than the audience, who may actually appreciate a moment to catch up [2].

12.1.5.6 Breath Control

Obviously, to speak implies the need to breathe first. If you breathe shallowly, your words will come out shallow. To be able to speak with a deep, confident tone, your breath needs to be similarly deep and full.

Therefore, be prepared to take a deep breath before you speak. A full lung gives you longer before you next need to breathe, giving you the chance to avoid a breath in the middle of a phrase. It also means you have the energy to complete a sentence without running out of steam and just trailing off.

Aim to breathe from the diaphragm. A proper deep breath makes the abdomen expand outwards and move back in as you breathe out. The diaphragm is the key muscle to control when you want to breathe efficiently [2].

12.2   Choice of Words

12.2.1 Useful Phrases to Use in Presentations

For a great many people, writing the content for a presentation and delivering it represents a considerable challenge. Moreover, there are many presenters who suffer from stage fright. Complicating all this is the fact that speeches in English are often delivered by non-native speakers. It is therefore beneficial if you have a stock of useful, correctly expressed phrases that can be adapted to the majority of presentations.

One advantage that a presenter has in this situation is that the formal structure of many presentations is similar and therefore many phrases can be re-used, to express a welcome to your listeners, to explain who another speaker is and the subject of the presentation, to lay out the outline, to summarise the key points or to ask for questions. The following sections offer some ways to accomplish each of these subtasks in a presentation. These kinds of pre-formed phrases help to guarantee that your presentation will be correctly and grammatically expressed [3].

12.2.1.1   Welcoming the Audience

Whenever a presentation is being given, the presenter should first make the audience feel welcome. The degree of formality used to express this thought is dictated by what relationship you already have with your audience. Here are a few suitable phrases:

> *Let me first say good morning (afternoon, evening) to you, ladies and gentlemen.*
> *I would like to say, on behalf of (the Ulusoy Clinic, etc.) how very welcome you are here today.*
> *Hello, everyone. Thanks for coming to the 7th Minor Procedures for your Beauty Seminar.*

12.2.1.2   Introducing Yourself, or the Person Who Is Going to Speak

As with the remarks indicating welcome, the level of formality needed in introducing yourself or someone else will depend on the audience to be addressed.

> *Allow me to say something about myself first. I am [Seckin Ulusoy] and today I will be discussing "Rejuvenating the Face" with you...*
> *Let me introduce myself before I begin. My name is Sinem Ulusoy. I am the marketing manager at Ulusoy Aesthetics Clinic.*
> *I'm Seckin from Ulusoy Aesthetics and I would like to tell you all about...*

12.2.1.3   Introducing the Topic

Following the welcome and the speaker saying who he/she is, it is important to outline the main topic of the presentation. This can be done in several ways:

My purpose today is to let you know about...
Today's topic is Facial Wrinkles" ...
I wish to take advantage of this meeting to discuss with you...
It gives me great pleasure to be able to talk to you about rhinoplasty...
I would like to give you a fairly brief overview on...
The presentation is going to cover the topic of...

12.2.1.4 Outlining the Objectives

It is always good to share your objectives with the audience at the beginning, as this makes it easier for them to follow the presentation and see where you are going with the material.

Today's objective is to...
My goal in presenting is for you to know about...

12.2.1.5 Structure

Once you have announced the topic and explained your presentation goals, you need to give the audience an idea of the structure you intend to follow. That way, they will have correct expectations from the talk.

Today's presentation consists of three parts...
We will begin by...
I will start by addressing,
I want to first discuss...
...following which, we will come onto...
...then there is...
...bringing us finally to the subject of...

12.2.1.6 First Section

With all these preliminary tasks accomplished, it is now time to begin the presentation proper. Here are a few suggestions on how to get started.

Let me begin by giving you some background on why...
I'd like to start with an explanation of...
First, let's take a quick look at how this subject first became so topical...
Now, before beginning, I would like to ask if anyone here knows when the first development on facial fillers began.
As I think you all know...
Even though nobody here is unfamiliar with the concept of neurotoxins, I wonder how many people could really define what it involves on the face?

12.2.1.7 Ending a Section

As you reach the end of a section in the presentation, let the audience know, so that they are aware a new subject is starting and do not lose their focus on the presentation.

That is about everything you need to know before a nose job, so let's move onto...
We have now learned the strategy of facial rejuvenation, so let's go to our next topic: Rhinoplasty.
So, that was the situation in 2010. Now...

12.2.1.8   Summing Up Part of a Presentation

It is vitally important to offer summaries of what you have discussed so far as you move through your presentation. Failure to do so usually means the audience immediately forgets what you have just been speaking about.

> *So, let's summarise what we have talked about so far…*
> *In a nutshell, here is what we can conclude at this point…*
> *Let's take a moment to recap what we have been discussing…*
> *Let me briefly reiterate what I have said so far.*
> *Before we move on, here's a short summary…*

12.2.1.9   Transitioning Between Topics

The following are all examples of how to manage the transition from one topic to another within a presentation.

> *I would like to now address another key area of concern…*
> *…which brings me nicely onto the next section, where we will discuss…*
> *Turning to the subject of…*
> *Let's move our focus onto…*

12.2.1.10   Giving Examples

It is common to need to illustrate your meaning by giving concrete examples. Here are some ways to do so.

> *Here is an example of that concept in action…*
> *I can show you a good example of that here…*
> *Let me illustrate what I mean by the following case study…*
> *Here is an illustration of my point…*
> *This brief case study will show you what I mean…*

12.2.1.11   Giving Details

It is common when presenting to need to supply more detailed information about particular points. These phrases help to signal that is what you are doing.

> *Let me provide a few more details on that issue…*
> *Allow me to give you a deeper insight into what's involved…*

12.2.1.12   Linking

It is often necessary to link one part of a presentation to another. Here are a few ways to do so.

> *Going back to my opening remarks…*
> *As I told you at the start of the presentation…*
> *You may recall, we said something similar when talking earlier about…*
> *This connects with the point touched on earlier, when I said…*

12.2.1.13   Referring Back to the Beginning

If a presentation is fairly lengthy, there is a danger that the audience lose track of the main topic and the aims of the presentation. One way to prevent this is to refer back occasionally to the beginning of the presentation.

> *Hopefully, we have now reached a point where you know more about...*
>> *Going back to where we started, we are now in a position to say...*
>> *As I finish this presentation, I would like to recap what was said at the very start...*
>> *If you remember what I said at the beginning, namely...you will hopefully now see how* *this proposed solution can help...*

12.2.1.14   Giving References for Information

It is very common in presentations to need to give references for specific information or facts you refer to. The following phrases can be used to state your sources:

> *On the basis of our own research...*
>> *A study undertaken in 1995 found that...*
>> *The data we collected make it clear that...*

12.2.1.15   Graphics and Images

Generally, presenters include many graphics and images in their slides. These are some ways to introduce different visual elements.

> *The best way to show that fact is with this graph.*
>> *Allow me to give you an illustration of how that actually looks...*
>> *This picture tells the whole story.*
>> *Looking at the graph, it is not difficult to see that...*
>> *If we refer to this table/graph/infographic, we can note how...*

12.2.1.16   Emphasising Key Points

To avoid a presentation beginning to be monotonous, it is important to highlight or emphasise particular points. The following are phrases you may wish to use.

> *It is important to emphasise that...*
>> *I especially want you to notice how...*
>> *A really key point is this:...*
>> *This is a really essential concept to grasp.*
>> *We must always remember this if we are to succeed in solving the issue.*

12.2.1.17   Expressing Yourself Differently

Sometimes, after explaining a point in one way, you may realise that the audience have not fully understood what you told them. In this situation, there is a need to paraphrase (express the same idea in different words). You can signal this is what you are doing by means of the following phrases.

> *To put it another way...*
>> *What I am saying is...*
>> *To put it in a nutshell.*
>> *Another way to put it is...*
>> *Or, in other words...*

12.2.1.18   Questions and Feedback

Audience questions are a highly valuable part of any presentation. Use the following expressions when handling questions or comments, or to ask for feedback.

Does anyone want to add anything at this point?
Now is a good time for us to look at any questions.
I am happy for you to interrupt if anything is unclear or you want to ask something.
Please don't be shy about asking questions. I will be happy to answer.
Let me know if you have any questions.
Would you like to clarify any points before we move on?
Unless there are any questions, we can go to our next topic…

12.2.1.19   Letting the Audience Know When to Ask Their Questions

If you take questions at the end of a presentation, there is no risk of the flow of the presentation being lost due to the need to follow up on questions asked as you go along. To signal that questions should be left until the end, you might try saying:

I have left time to address your questions at the end of my talk.
Please keep your questions until the end, where I will be very happy to answer them.
Could I please ask you to give your comments at the end?

12.2.1.20   Checking You Have Given the Right Answer

When a question comes from the audience, it is important to make sure you have understood what the individual really wants to know. Check that your answer was adequate in the following ways:

Is that the kind of information you were looking for?
Was I able to answer your question?
Hopefully, that answers your enquiry.

12.2.1.21   When You Do Not Have an Answer

On occasion, you may not be in a position to answer a question coming from the audience. This need not be a major issue. However, it is best to acknowledge the situation.

A very good point that I will need to look into before I can give you a real answer. Let me get back to you.
Unfortunately, I don't have that information at present, but if you let me, I will answer that after I check some facts.
That is an interesting question. I do not know what to say. What are your thoughts?
Your question is very interesting and something I would like to know, too. Unfortunately, the data we have are not adequate at the moment to provide a definitive answer.
I am afraid I am not the right person to answer that question, but many thanks for asking anyway.

12.2.1.22   Summarising and Concluding

Use the end of your presentation as an opportunity to reiterate the key messages of the presentation. You might say:

Allow me to conclude by reminding you what we discussed...
To conclude, here is a summary of the key learning points.
After examining both the advantages and disadvantages, I conclude...
So, that is the end of what I wanted to say today. Many thanks for attending.
Thanks to everyone for listening. I have enjoyed being able to speak to you.
That concludes my talk. Thank you.
We have now reached the end, so it only remains to thank you for your kind attention.

12.2.1.23 Handing on to Another Presenter

In situations where you are not the last speaker, it may be helpful to use some of the following expressions:

Now I will hand over to your other speaker for today, Dr Seckin Ulusoy from Istanbul University.
Ok, Marina, I am handing over to you now.

12.3 What to Wear When Presenting

It is abundantly clear from the feedback received from multiple presentations that the choice of what to wear has a major bearing on whether the presenter achieves a high level of credibility or not. A well-dressed presenter usually commands more attention from an audience and is better listened to. Despite this fact, many presenters fail to plan adequately what they will wear to present [4].

Nobody wants the delivery of their presentation to be undermined by wearing shabby-looking clothes or having an inappropriate dress style. The following are seven key points for presenters to bear in mind when choosing what to wear [4].

Your dress style should be a little smarter than your audience Consider who will attend your presentation and how they tend to be dressed. This will then guide how you dress. If your appearance is somewhat smarter than the audience, they will tend to place greater trust in what you are saying. Wearing a jacket typically makes an outfit seem smarter.

Ensure you choose a well-fitting outfit Even if an item of clothing is very high quality, if it does not fit properly, it will detract from your appearance. In a presentation, the audience are all looking towards the presenter, hence ill-fitting clothing is easily noticed and may become what your listeners focus on. The audience notice a bulging button that is about to pop. When your trousers are too short, people will notice your ankles. If the fit of your outfit is an issue, get the items modified to fit by a tailor.

Be alert to the best choice of colour Dark colours generally make a presenter appear better than light colours. Nonetheless, wearing a lighter colour may convey a warmer impression and is often better suited to a presentation in a warmer country or location. It is also a good idea, where possible, to check what colour the background (walls or curtain, etc.) will be. Although many venues have light-coloured décor, this may not be the case. It would make a suboptimal impression if the colour of your outfit fitted the background to the extent that your body seems to be disappearing.

Avoid appearing "over the top" Female presenters should be careful with outfits that reveal a large amount of cleavage, as they may detract from the presenter's credibility. Likewise outfits that expose the upper leg. Although such outfits definitely grab the audience's attention, they may ruin a presentation if the outfit upstages the presenter. For skirts, knee length is more suitable than a mini-skirt.

Accessories are also important The addition of accessories can make an outfit even more appealing, but care needs to be taken that the accessory is not all your audience can focus on. When speaking, avoid toying with a necklace or constantly adjusting your cufflinks. Remove your name tag as you present. The audience should already know who you are from your introduction and a name tag rarely improves the appearance of an outfit.

Be well-groomed Everything you do should make the audience attend to the presentation, rather than to flaws in your personal grooming or hygiene. A jacket with a snow shower of dandruff, dirty spectacles and food stuck between your teeth all tend to distract attention away from your message. This is especially the case when you are very near to your audience, as in small group presentations. Shoes are something that most people notice immediately. Ensure they are clean, well-polished and do not have big holes in them.

Be careful about how you stand Stand straight, with your shoulders held back. Even the snappiest outfit in the world will fail to look good if the wearer is slouching or leaning whilst presenting.

12.4 Presenter's Attitude

It is one thing to know what makes a person successful, but quite another to actually implement the changes needed to achieve success. Filling this gap between knowledge of what to do and actual improved performance is what gives an opportunity to particular individuals to be an elite presenter [5].

12.4.1 So, What Makes a Presenter Highly Successful?

There are four principal factors which mark out speakers of exceptional ability, namely [5]:

1. The presentations they deliver contain messages that are relevant, affect individuals and are strongly persuasive.
2. They are not frightened to challenge audiences to think and develop their intellectual and emotional capacities.
3. They give wise messages clearly, in a way that people find really convincing.
4. They can change not just how people think, but also how they act.

It is a common misconception that possession of these abilities is something only truly elite presenters should strive for [5]. On the contrary, every presenter should aim to increase their skills in this way.

In fact, whatever the nature of the presentation, whether it is a monthly team briefing, an update on a project, a sales presentation or something else altogether, it is highly valuable to attempt to emulate the techniques of great presenters, especially those who deliver motivational speeches.

Of course, for some presentations, the primary objective may not involve motivating change, but even so, every presenter would ideally wish to [5]:

- Fascinate the audience from the very beginning and keep them enthralled throughout the presentation.
- Connect with the audience on both an intellectual and emotional level.
- Ensure that the message and the presenter remain lodged in the audience's memory.
- Maintain engagement, curiosity and trust in the presentation.
- Inspire the listeners to take action after the presentation.

Start a presentation with a story that conveys a powerful and pertinent message and which has relevance to the entire audience.

Truly elite presenters do not just relate an anecdote, but rather make the audience re-live the experience through their use of acting. For example, if the character in a story acted angrily, the presenter makes the audience feel this anger in her words. As she expresses sadness, she seems almost about to cry herself.

Effective presenters also deliberately get in amongst the audience members and engage in as much eye contact as possible.

An effective technique that great presenters often use is to group things into threes when speaking. For example, she may refer to "courage, dedication and determination".

Any story usually benefits from the injection of a humorous element, as long as it is appropriate.

The facial expression and body language of effective presenters are carefully matched to the words used in the presentation.

Vocal tone is always clearly audible, although there is variation and at times a quiet tone is adopted, to draw the audience into confidence with the speaker.

Effective speakers often ask rhetorical questions that have a personal resonance for audience members: "Why do managers who make their employees unhappy often seem unhappy themselves?" As the audience begins to notice the same thing, a follow-up question gets them to nod a second time in agreement: "And why are those miserable managers the same ones who always complain about a lack of enthusiasm in new starters?"

This sharing of common experience is one of the most fruitful ways to establish a connection with an audience. For this reason, such questions are commonly put at the beginning of a presentation, when the speaker is establishing rapport with the audience. By meticulously choreographing their own performance in the first few minutes of a presentation, speakers can get the audience engaged and convey that they are people who are both likeable and trustworthy [5].

12.5 Timing Your Presentation

12.5.1 What Is the Optimal Number of Slides?

Previously, it used to be stated that an optimal number of slides in a presentation could be calculated on the basis of one slide each minute. Nowadays, however, the consensus is that this is an over-simplification.

There are several factors to consider. One factor is how complex the material is. Another consideration is whether there is a complex graphic or large amount of text to be covered. Build slides (where the content is gradually revealed) are slower than standard slides, sometimes significantly so. Therefore, in 30 min, the range for slide numbers may extend from around 10 (for complex slides) to approximately 150 (for less content-rich slides).

12.5.2 Assess How Complex Your Content Is

It is vital to think about how complicated the message of your presentation is, and how easily audiences will be able to understand it.

It is fair to say, however, that a slide should generally take at least 30 s to present. If you can present it in less time, it may be better to combine the material from that slide with another, possibly as an element in a build slide. For example, if you wanted to highlight several elements on a diagram, it would be more efficient and less distracting to ensure you used one slide rather than several. You can progressively build up the labels on the slide. This is generally the case when you are discussing the same main idea on several slides. If you keep presenting slides in less than 30 s, your audience may have the sense that you are rushing over key details in an attempt to finish quickly.

In contrast, where a slide contains complicated concepts or has a large volume of text, even 1 min to present may be insufficient. For a highly technical presentation, it is usually appropriate to spend between 1.5 and 3 min presenting a slide with a key concept. If the slide cannot be comfortably presented in under 3.5 min, the material would often be better divided into two or more slides. Another possibility may be to use a build slide (or several).

Thus, the one slide per minute rule of thumb is inapplicable in many cases and it is usually more advisable to plan the number of slides on the basis of how complex the material is, how the ideas are separate from each other and what makes it easiest for the audience to understand.

12.5.3 Assess How Long You Need for Each Idea

To plan how long you may spend on each section, first assume that it will take up around 15% of the time to present the introduction and conclusion. The remaining 85% can then be divided by the number of principal points you need to cover, giving a fair estimate of how long you can afford to spare on each point, assuming all the points are of equal weight.

To take a practical example, if you have a 20-min slot to present, you can allocate around 3 min for your introduction and conclusion. That leaves 17 min. If you have eleven key points to make, you may spend 1.5 min on each ($17/11 \approx 1.5$). The introduction and conclusion should involve an absolute maximum of six slides, whereas there will probably be between 10 and 14 slides for the main body of the presentation.

Or, suppose you have a rather longer slot available, say 1 h. The beginning and conclusion take up around 9 min (15% of 60 min is 9 min). That leaves 51 min. If you want to present seven main ideas, you have around 7 min for each key point ($51/7 = 7$ min, with 2 min to spare). You can then work out how many slides should be created on the basis of how complex each key point is.

12.5.4 Now Decide on Timing Within Each Section

If a presentation will last more than a few minutes, it is also worth timing each sub-section of the presentation. In the example above, if the first idea consists of five sub-sections, you can reasonably allocate just under 1.5 min to each (since $7/5 = 1.4$). Obviously, this calculation assumes each subsection is of equal weight, which may not actually be the case.

The method outlined above is a more effective way to decide on the timing and to calculate how many slides to include than a rule of thumb such as "one slide per minute". Once the slides have been put together, you will need to practise and adapt the timing, depending on the complexity of the material and how easy it is to present.

12.5.5 Add Up the Different Types of Slides

Some experts recommend classifying slides in a presentation into different categories, such as "short", "medium" and "long". Short slides, for example, take around 30 s to explain, medium slides around 1 min and long slides up to 3 min. When the slides have been classified in this way, it is easier to estimate the total length of time needed to present the set.

Nonetheless, it is only by performing a full rehearsal of the presentation that presenters can gain an accurate idea of exactly how long it takes to deliver the entire presentation. Be sure to use a stopwatch to get an objective view of the situation.

There is often a discrepancy between the length of delivery in a rehearsal and at an actual presentation event. This may relate to how anxious the presenter feels and what level of energy they can put into the presentation. When planning, try to factor this difference into your timing calculations.

12.5.6 Set Timings for Different Sections

The final stage of preparation is to define timing points for specific points in the presentation, such that you can be aware quickly of any timing issues before you over-run. In a 1-h presentation, for example, you should note down which slide to reach after 10 min, half an hour and 10 min before the end.

These timings are helpful in indicating whether a presenter is moving too quickly or too slowly. If, for example, you fall behind schedule, you can skip over some material that is not essential to the key message. Conversely, if you find yourself ahead of schedule, you might want to offer the audience an extra chance to ask questions before you reach the conclusion. The timings can help ensure your presentation fits neatly into its slot.

The timings technique is very versatile and is widely used by expert presenters. It is best to actually write down the times, along with when you want to be finished. The time to finish should ideally be no closer than 5 min to the next speaker, if you are in a conference. Remember to allow for the fact that few presentations actually start on time, as many audience members arrive late.

When you know the timing for each section, you can work out the time at which you need to reach specific sections in the presentation. If section one plus the introduction take 14 min, and you start at 10:04 am, you will need to get there at 10:18 am [6].

12.5.7 Be Careful to Check Twice

It is worth adding a note here to suggest you double check any timing calculations. Presenters are often somewhat nervous on the day of the presentation, and it is easy to miscalculate the timings. Speaking from bitter experience, I can say that a miscalculation can easily mean you end up having to omit important sections in order to finish on time.

In summary, then, timing along with tone of voice, attitude, and dress style are all elements that every presenter should pay careful attention to. By getting these aspects right, you greatly enhance the success of any type of presentation.

References

1. The importance of tone of voice and why you should get it right. https://www.pixus.uk/the-importance-of-tone-of-voice-and-why-you-should-get-it-right/. Accessed 24 Oct 2021.
2. Your voice during a presentation. Syntaxis. https://www.syntaxis.com/your-voice-during-a-presentation. Accessed 4 Oct 2021.
3. Useful English phrases for a presentation. 2 Oct 2017. https://www.topcorrect.com/blog/useful-english-phrases-for-a-presentation/. Accessed 4 Oct 2021.
4. Pachter B. Dressing for a presentation? Choose your clothing wisely. https://www.linkedin.com/pulse/dressing-presentation-choose-your-clothing-wisely-barbara-pachter/. Accessed 4 Oct 2021.
5. Maurice D. No.1 presentation tip: 'attitude makes all the difference'. 21 April 2016. https://mindfulpresenter.com/presentation-tip-attitude/. Accessed 4 Oct 2021.
6. Marshall LB. How to time a presentation. https://www.quickanddirtytips.com/business-career/public-speaking/how-to-time-a-presentation.

13.1 What Is Body Language?

It is very normal for presenters to feel apprehensive when they are about to speak. Presenters are there to get the undivided focus of the entire audience, after all. However, to present successfully, you should project an air of feeling relaxed and confident in what you are saying. Body language can help to convey this impression. Your dress style, the position you stand in, how you walk, the expression on your face and how you move your hands and arms all constitute what is termed "body language".

Body language plays an equal, if not greater, role in communication than verbal language (i.e. the words you speak). Indeed, even before you open your mouth, your body has already begun to communicate with the audience.

Actors are experts in the skilful use of body language. Acting on stage or on the screen involves the constant use of elements of body language to convey a character's personality, that person's emotions and passions and the reaction to the unfolding drama. It is worth studying how they achieve this and emulating their techniques.

Thus, presenters should see mastery of body language as a highly potent and beneficial skill that assists in getting their message across whenever they present.

13.2 Advice on Using Body Language to Your Advantage

1. **The First Messages Come from Your Appearance:** Ensure that you have chosen a suitable outfit to wear and pay close attention to your personal grooming (hair, shaving, make-up, etc.) If your outfit makes you look like a slob or a spiv, your audience will assume that is your real character.

2. **Remember to Smile:** As you come into the room, or whilst someone introduces you, give a warm smile to the people around. Make your smile convey warmth and sincerity. It is normal to be quite anxious before speaking, but

                                                     149
C. C. Cingi et al., *Improving Online Presentations*,
https://doi.org/10.1007/978-3-031-28328-4_13

conquer your nerves, stand tall and keep calm and collected. This is the point when your audience are forming the all-important first impression.

3. **Avoid Leaning on the Lecture Stand or Using It for Support:** Presenters who cling to the podium convey the unfortunate impression that they are scared and lack strength.

4. **Keep a Slight Smile on Your Face as You Start the Introduction:** As the presentation moves on, you can adopt a somewhat more serious facial expression.

5. **Do Not Wag Your Finger Towards the Audience:** Pointing a finger comes across as rude and hostile. When showing your hands, keep them palms upward and apart, which usually conveys a much warmer and more positive emotion.

6. **From Time to Time, Gesticulate With Your Arms:** The arms can help you emphasise particularly significant parts of your speech, but be careful not to overdo it as this rapidly becomes distracting and may make the message harder to understand. Use sparingly to get the maximum effect.

7. **Keep Your Eyes on the Audience:** Try to establish eye contact with as many members of the audience as possible. Avoid the situation where you only engage a single person in eye contact. Look at the audience as though they were individuals, not just a part of a crowd. Failure to establish eye contact makes a presenter seem untrustworthy.

8. **Avoid Pacing Up and Down:** Whilst walking up and down the stage can help the speaker feel more relaxed, for the audience, this becomes highly distracting. It is certainly not necessary to remain rooted to the spot but walking to somewhere else on the stage should be for emphasis or variety, and accordingly should not be constant.

9. **Make Use of Your Head and Face:** Presenters can emphasise a particular point by moving their head or changing facial expression. Shake the head whilst emphasising a thing to avoid. Nod in approval as you offer some tip or piece of advice. The eyebrows can be raised or you might remove your spectacles, if you want to draw attention to one particular point.

10. **Manage your Voice:** You should speak at a moderate pace, articulating your words carefully. Slowing down helps to emphasise a certain point. Repetition, yes, repetition, helps to highlight an issue. Try explaining the same idea in different words. Alter the volume of your voice for emphasis. Occasional silence is also an excellent way to focus the audience's attention. Say your point, then pause in silence to let it sink in, before continuing [1–3].

13.3   Ways for Presenters to Utilise Body Language

Effective use of body language can transform a relatively uninspiring presentation without movement into one full of dynamism, with the audience fully engaged and listening. Body language involves multiple elements, but can be categorised under five main headings [1]:

- Face expressions
- Eye contact
- Posture
- Gesture
- Movement and position

Although the analysis of body language involves many small details, these details have a disproportionately large influence on how your presentation is perceived. If your body language mirrors the messages of your presentation and your tone of voice, you will be guaranteed to be more effective and persuasive [1–3].

13.3.1 Face Expression

The expression "face-to-face" indicates clearly the importance of facial expression when people meet each other. The facial expressions play a major role in how we communicate. Ordinarily, the expression on our faces is something we may not consciously attend to; however, in certain situations, e.g. during delivery of a presentation, it is helpful to attend to what message our facial expressions may be sending.

The initial and absolutely essential step in controlling facial expression is to check that you *are* actually expressing yourself through facial expression. Too often, a presenter delivers a speech with a blank expression on his or her face. This is the body language equivalent of speaking in a monotone, and the effect is similar—the audience will be bored and immediately stop listening. Even a very minimal amount of facial expression, such as keeping the eyes wide open, smiling or raising an eyebrow, is an enormous improvement on expressionless delivery. At particular intervals, presenters can check themselves to ensure they have not fallen back into a blank look and can consciously adjust their facial expression.

However, facial expressions need to appear natural to be effective. If you simply memorise where to smile or raise your eyebrows, the effect will be lost completely. You need to think about the message you are giving, and your facial expressions should reflect that message. When the facial expressions are congruent with the content, not only is the content easier to understand, but the audience will view you as more honest in what you are saying. Never forget that facial expression plays a big part in how trustworthy people find each other. It is also important to think about how far away from you the audience is sitting. People sitting a long way from the back will not see subtle changes in facial expression. This means expressions may need to be made more obvious than in everyday life [1].

13.3.2 Eye Contact

Facial expressions in general are important, but there is one aspect of facial movement that is especially important—making eye contact with your audience.

As with all expressions of body language in a presentation setting, the size of the venue and the number of people you will be addressing have an important impact on the way you will use eye contact. There are, however, some principles which apply virtually everywhere, as follows.

Try to engage each audience member in eye contact on more than one occasion If presenters always look in the same direction, the audience will find the presentation uninteresting and tedious. They will not feel part of the event. To avoid this, presenters should look around the room, making eye contact with everyone, provided the audience is not too large. If it is a very large group, presenters should at least look towards every section of the audience on several occasions.

Eye contact is not something to fear The reason intense eye contact can unnerve people is because it evokes a strong emotional response. Staring someone in the eyes for too long can come across as a very hostile act. Eye contact in presentations is not of this type. When you briefly establish eye contact with audience members, the message they receive is that you are wanting to check they are able to understand the presentation. It shows you value their involvement. So, whilst it might seem easier to fix your gaze on an empty spot, if you do so, the audience may well feel their involvement is not valued or appreciated.

Eye contact needs to be the right kind So, eye contact is generally beneficial, but needs to be brief and not come across as a piercing stare. Keep your eyes moving from individual to individual and from group to group.

Keep in mind that eye contact will be established in various ways, depending on the situation. The important practice point is that eye contact should be made in presentations if you want the audience to feel involved and therefore become fully engaged [1].

13.3.3 Posture

After thinking about how to express yourself facially and the importance of eye contact, we now move on to consider posture. Posture refers to the way a person holds his or her body. The way a presenter sits or stands during a presentation has an enormous effect on the way the presenter and the presentation are perceived. Posture sends a message long before any verbal communication begins.

Given the importance of posture, the following are some key pieces of advice:

- **Avoid Slouching:** Whenever you present, you should hold yourself upright and in an open posture. This posture conveys the impression of confidence and appears welcoming to the audience. Adopting such a posture also helps the presenter to feel more confident. If you have a tendency to slouch, the audience will perceive that you do not attach importance to the presentation. This will then mean they are not going to attend carefully to what you have to say, either.

- **Try Not to Appear Tense:** To present well, you need to feel relaxed and to convey that impression to the audience. An upright posture characterised by rigidity does not appear relaxed. Even if in truth you are quite anxious talking to an audience, you cannot convey this impression and still hope to get them to trust you. Before you start to speak, pause a moment and breathe deeply. At intervals in the presentation, keep thinking about the need to avoid seeming tense. When you pause and breathe deeply for a moment, this has the additional benefit of letting your audience catch up with the presentation. During the brief pause, make a conscious effort to dispel your tension and adjust the way you hold yourself, as well as your facial expression.
- **Consider Who the Audience Are:** There is a world of difference between presenting to the executive committee of an international company and talking with a class of young kindergarteners. An upright posture is appropriate in every setting, but the level of formality called for differs considerably. Think, for example, about how you intend to handle questions. Should they be kept for the end, or can you take questions as you go along? Your posture sends a clear message about how open you are to audience interaction.
- **Adaptability Is Important:** If you present from a sitting position or from behind a lecture stand, do not cling to the chair or stand and avoid using a stand as a shield. Presenters need to have an open posture and communicate openly, whatever the situation is. If you present to a large audience, there may only be one fixed microphone, which will constrain your movement on the stage. If you need to hold a microphone that also imposes limitations on the ability to gesture. In an ideal world, the presenter knows these things in advance, but in reality presenters often face unexpected challenges and there is a need for flexibility [1].

13.3.4 Gestures

Plenty of facial expression, eye contact and excellent posture are certainly key elements in presenting successfully; however, if your arms remain perfectly immobile, the effect will be extremely disconcerting. Of course, the opposite case, where the presenter gesticulates wildly, like a character in a comedy film, is equally inappropriate.

What is needed is something in-between. Gestures should be used to clarify your point and to add variety. To achieve this purpose, gestures should be relevant. So, to give an example, if you want to emphasise the difference between a very low number and a very high number, you can indicate this by showing a low and a high level with your arms and the side of your hand. When going through five reasons, try numbering the reasons off on your fingers. You might also want to gesture towards the audience to emphasise they are included. In the latter case, however, it is important not to point, as this can come across as hostile or accusatory. You can also gesture to indicate features shown on a slide, such as a trend on a graph. Furthermore, if you are working towards the climax of your presentation, you may need to gradually increase the amount of gesturing you do, so that the key messages you want the audience to take home are clearly signalled through body language.

There is some valuable detailed information about gesturing with your hands on the Science of People website [2]. In any case, whatever gestures you employ need to appear spontaneous and comfortable. One way to ensure your gestures appear this way is to practise often. You can film yourself, then critique your performance afterwards. Alternatively, it is worth asking friends or colleagues for their comments. In the same way that other features of body language, such as eye contact and facial expression, need to be modified depending on how large the audience and the venue are, so gestures will require similar adaptation to the circumstances [1].

13.3.5 Where to Stand and Move

The final aspect of body language to consider, position and movement, requires a varied approach, depending on the venue and setup. It is generally easy to work out whether you will be able to move around for a presentation or need to remain in one position; however, it is prudent to assess your options in advance.

Thus, in a setting where you have a large stage from which to present, being able to move from one part of the stage to another makes the presentation more interesting visually and increases engagement with different sections of your audience. In a similar way, if presenters wish to interact directly with the audience, they may move to the front of the stage to ask a question or pose a challenge, so that they can observe more closely how the audience reacts. This helps the presenter and makes the audience feel the presenter is more interested in them. After all, there is a huge difference in perception between being addressed (where the individual person receives a message) and being lectured at (where the audience are just a group). Audiences want to feel their opinion also counts. In any case, movement on the stage should never come across as idle wandering. It should serve a definite purpose and appear logical in intent.

To conclude, body language consists of the five elements outlined above. It is a powerful language, which, when used appropriately, reinforces your message. It clarifies the meaning and increases audience engagement. However, body language should never be seen as an optional extra to a presentation. It needs to be co-ordinated with the content and tone of the presentation, so that maximum impact can be achieved. Keep practising and remember to enjoy the experience of presenting [1].

References

1. How to use body language during a presentation. 19 Feb 2018. https://etonx.com/how-to-use-body-language-during-a-presentation/. Accessed 4 Oct 2021.

2. 60 hand gestures you should be using and their meaning. https://www.scienceofpeople.com/hand-gestures/. Accessed 30 Nov 2021.
3. 10 body language tips for presentations. https://www.englishclub.com/business-english/body-language.php. Accessed 4 Oct 2021.

14.1   Utilisation of Visual Elements When Presenting

Visuals can potentially strengthen the audience's ability to understand the subject of your presentation, to clarify particular points, to add to your impact as a presenter and to generate more enthusiasm in your listeners.

The term "visuals" refers to any material of a visual nature, which includes graphics, photographic images, video clips, animations and so on. The choice of visuals is dictated by the intended purpose. Some reasons why you may wish to include visuals are [1]

- To provide a visual summary.
- To replace a lengthy piece of spoken text, such as when showing a graph instead of giving each piece of data separately.
- To provide a specific example that makes a concept clearer.
- To present a striking image that produces greater impact than telling the same idea. For example, if you wanted to describe the effect of excessive alcohol use on the liver, you might share an image of a cirrhosed liver next to a healthy liver. A visual used like this may be used to generate different audience emotions—anger, shock, fear, etc.
- To underline your spoken message.
- To make a point easier to remember for the audience.
- To give solid evidence that enhances your credibility as a presenter.
- To get the audience engaged and keep them focused.
- To facilitate audience understanding [1].

C. C. Cingi et al., *Improving Online Presentations*,
https://doi.org/10.1007/978-3-031-28328-4_14

14.1.1 Preparing and Utilising Visuals

Having identified a part in a presentation where a visual is suitable, presenters should first ensure that the visual can be readily understood at a glance by the audience. Clarity is vitally important. Whilst visuals may be used at any point in a presentation, they are best reserved to emphasise key messages. Too many visuals can put a strain on audiences.

14.1.1.1   Getting Prepared

- Consider in what way the visual adds to your message. What reaction are you hoping for from the audience?
- Visuals should fit in with the general flow of the presentation, otherwise they become distracting.
- Keep images uncluttered to avoid becoming confused or unclear.
- All visuals should be high quality, clear and focused on the subject.
- The overall graphical style should maintain consistency in terms of fonts used, colour scheme and slide layout.
- Data are best presented graphically, in charts, for example.
- Do not force your audience both to read and slide and listen to you speaking simultaneously. The visual should emphasise what you are already saying.
- Each visual should be focused on one principal message.
- Do not overdo the visuals. Use sparingly to offer support and illustration of key points, not for decoration.
- Plan in such a way that if the visuals become unusable, such as due to a power cut, the presentation still makes sense on its own.
- Before the actual presentation, practise delivery, including showing the visuals, and solicit the opinion of peers, friends or colleagues on whether the visual is clear and what message they think it sends.

14.1.1.2   At the Time of Presentation

- Make sure all the audience members get a clear view of any visuals.
- Presenters should be facing the audience, not the visuals.
- Never read straight off the visual.
- Once a visual is displayed, the audience will be entirely focused on that. Your speech needs to be about the visual. If you talk about something other than the visual, the audience will not pay attention to you.
- The audience should be told what the visual is for.
- After you have explained the visual, stop displaying it.

14.1.1.3   Fit the Presentation to Your Target Audience

The choice of visuals is something to approach carefully. You will need images of a kind that speak clearly to the audience. Visuals should reflect your audience's tastes and be of things they find familiar. If you are talking about food to an Italian audience, Chinese bird nest soup is a less effective visual than a plate of steaming tagliatelle. Consider in addition what type of visual is suited to the occasion.

Humorous cartoon images are suitable if the event is relatively light-hearted. Conversely, more serious or formal events call for more sober-looking illustrations [1].

14.1.2 Different Kinds of Visuals

Since visuals are available in a wide range of different types, presenters need to ascertain the most suitable type for the event and the expected audience.

14.1.2.1 PowerPoint

Use of Microsoft PowerPoint has become very widespread, thanks to its user-friendly interface, which allows visually appealing and professional-looking presentations to be created easily and lets the user incorporate or modify other material into a presentation in a straightforward manner. Including visuals in a PowerPoint slide set helps to focus the attention of your audience. Projected PowerPoint slides are often easier to see than other forms of projection (such as writing on transparencies), and presenters can display the slides behind themselves whilst facing the audience. This means the audience can see both the presenter's visual expression and the slides at the same time. Despite its many advantages, however, this application can still produce poor results if the task of preparing slides is not undertaken in a professional way.

Tips
- Use a relatively plain, uncluttered background for your slides.
- Keep to a limited number of different font faces and sizes.
- If you decide to use an animation, this should only be where it helps with understanding. An animation is good to show a dynamic process. Avoid using animations for pure entertainment purposes—it looks unprofessional.
- Employ a size of font that is clearly legible on projection, i.e. minimum 24 points.
- Present lists as bullet points.
- If a diagram is complicated, it may be best to provide printed copies of the diagram to the audience as these copies can be more easily examined.
- Do not overload slides with text.
- Red and green text is hard to read and many people are red-green colour blind, therefore avoid this combination where possible.
- Each slide should contain a single main message.
- Be prepared for technical failure (system down, power cut, etc.) by knowing how to present without the benefit of visuals. A poster or handouts are a reasonable backup [1].

14.1.2.2 Whiteboards

If a presenter needs to add some extra details to a presentation during delivery, such as explaining a concept in more detail, illustrating how a process works or breaking down a technical term, a whiteboard is often the best place to do so. Furthermore, whiteboards can be used for recording audience questions or answers. By having a whiteboard on display, important information that needs to be referenced several times, such as a formula or definition, can be easily seen by the audience whenever they need to be reminded.

Advice:
- Do not be too quick to erase the whiteboard since audiences are often slow writing down their notes.
- Be brief, to avoid turning away from the audience for lengthy periods.
- Keep handwriting clear and of sufficient size to be seen.
- It is worth practising writing on the whiteboard in advance to deal with any nervousness you may have writing in front of an audience [1].

14.1.2.3   Handouts

A handout is usually a printed set of notes to distribute to the audience. This document usually repeats key information from the presentation and may give more detailed data in some topics, so that the presenter does not overburden the audience with more information than they can comfortably understand in one go.

Advice
- It is essential to plan the timing of giving out your handouts
- If you distribute the handout at the start or during the presentation, there is a risk the audience may read the handout instead of listening to the presentation. They may feel they already know what you are going to say.
- Conversely, if you only distribute the handout at the end of the presentation, the audience may have spent an unnecessary time trying to take notes, when they may have profited more by just listening carefully.

One solution to this dilemma is to supply a handout at the start, but one where there are a number of gaps that the audience need to fill in by listening to the presentation. The handout can certainly include any graphs or charts since they are generally easier to see properly in printed form than when projected onto a screen [1].

14.1.2.4   Including Video in a Presentation

The inclusion of video clips in a presentation is an effective way to increase engagement by the audience and generate enthusiasm for the topic. Videos offer movement, visual variety and audio to a presentation.

Advice on using video:
- Make sure that any video clips do actually reinforce the message of the presentation.
- The duration should be only as long as absolutely essential.
- Lengthy clips must always be avoided.

- Since video clips may interrupt the continuity of any presentation, it is vital to inform the audience of the reason for including the clip and explain what you wish them to notice.
- Tell the audience how long the clip lasts in advance of showing it.

14.1.2.5   Using a Flip Chart

Flip charts offer a very cost-effective and non-technology-dependent way to add extra information during the course of a presentation. They are particularly useful if you have a small audience and want to do some brainstorming for ideas with the group. Just as with a whiteboard, a flip chart can be used to summarise information or to continuously show some key information needed to make sense of a presentation.

Advice on using a flip chart:
- Prior to delivering your presentation, position the flip chart where it is easy to use.
- Do some preparation of the flip chart in advance, such as adding key headings. This will save time.
- The flip chart can be positioned in such a way that you can write on it at the same time as facing towards the audience.
- Each sheet of the flip chart should carry just one principal idea.
- Write in a legible way. Handwriting should be large and capital letters may be easier to read.
- Ask your audience if they can easily see your handwriting. A flip chart is not helpful if an audience exceeds a certain size.
- Most of the writing should be in black or blue, with red ink used to highlight particular words or phrases.
- You can pencil in notes lightly on the flip chart in advance and rule lines for your own benefit. Audiences cannot see these small notes, but they help you keep everything organised.
- You can flip back over previous sheets to reiterate and reinforce a message.
- As with using a whiteboard, it may be helpful to practise writing on the flip chart before the presentation, so that nerves do not get the better of you [1].

14.1.2.6   Posters

Posters can be assembled from several different visuals, e.g. graphical representations or images. Posters are typically straightforward to carry around and can be made to any degree of complexity desired. There is a significant cost to producing very complicated posters, however.

Advice on posters:
- A poster should have a single key message or theme.
- It should be colourful.
- Write titles with BLOCK CAPITALS.

- Posters are unsuitable as a presentation aid where there are many people in an audience since those at the back cannot clearly see the poster [1].

14.1.2.7   Use of Props: Products, Objects, etc.

Props have the advantage that they add interest and may increase the impact of a presentation. In certain types of presentation, such as an experimental demonstration, they are indispensable.

Advice on using props:

- If your audience is a small group, you can let the audience members handle certain objects. However, be careful that they are not distracted by the prop to the extent of ignoring the rest of the presentation.
- For larger groups, you can carry the prop from section to section for everyone to view.
- Once you start showing a prop, the audience will concentrate on it rather than you. Therefore, avoiding revealing the object before you have supplied any background needed to appreciate what it is.
- Give the reasons for showing the prop.
- For demonstration of a product or a scientific experiment, your actions should be very clear. Move more slowly than usual and with greater emphasis. Give a commentary on the actions you are performing [1].

14.1.3 Important Factors to Consider in the Use of Visuals

Endeavour to ascertain in advance the layout of the venue where you are to present. Check how the room is equipped and ensure that any visuals you intend to use will be suitable for the venue. However, do not rely on everything working as expected. You should always prepare a backup plan. If you do show any visuals, ideally the audience should be able to take in the key message at a glance [1].

14.1.3.1   Practising

Prior to the actual event, be sure to practise using the equipment you need to project any visuals, so that you can iron out any technical hitches. This practise will be invaluable if something goes wrong on the day of the presentation.

14.1.3.2   Utilise Colour

It has been discovered by researchers that utilisation of colour is associated with higher levels of enthusiasm for reading an article or attending a presentation. Fortunately, most presentation software offers the ability to create colourful slides and visuals.

When planning a colour scheme to use, it is helpful to employ a colour wheel. The following are factors to consider [1]:

- Complementary colours are located on opposite sides of the wheel. Because the use of complementary colours increases contrast, text in a complementary colour to the background is more legible.
- Adjacent colours are considered analogous and instil a sense of harmony. A colour scheme using analogous colours helps the presentation seem more coherent.
- Keep to a relatively limited palate of colours to avoid appearing amateurish. You should also aim for consistency in the use of colours. For example, highlighted words should appear in the same colour on every slide. Bear in mind that certain colour combinations have particular connotations in specific cultures. Purple is said to symbolise evil in Japan, for instance. If possible, harmonise the colours with the message you wish to send.
- Since many people have an innate inability to see the difference between blue and green or red and green, these colours should not be used for contrast in figures. Where such colours occur next to each other naturally, make sure there are textual labels to clarify which is which [1].

14.2 Presenting Positively

Whilst positivity may be applied to virtually any kind of communication, there are plenty of communication scenarios where positivity is either irrelevant or inappropriate. However, in the great majority of presentations, the objective is to put forward a proposal, persuade the audience or advocate for a specific viewpoint [2]. In these circumstances, positivity is a very necessary component of an effective presentation.

14.2.1 Choice of Words

It is not a surprising conclusion to learn that the choice of words used when delivering a presentation has a vital impact on the effectiveness of that presentation. However, a more subtle point is that putting a positive spin on the words and phrases you use can increase the strength of the communication channel linking the presenter and audience. To achieve this kind of positive spin, there is a need to think about three key aspects:

Firstly, Decide How Much Positivity to Inject: Consider whether you are aiming to be evangelical in tone or to strike a more down-to-earth, yet still enthusiastic, note. At this stage, the exact choice of particular words is not important since you are concentrating on the overall tone.

Secondly, Try to Avoid Words with a Negative Connotation: The simple rule to follow is to reword any sentences containing the words with a negative connotation into a sentence using the corresponding positive words, as follows [2]:

Negative-Sounding Words: but, however, they, them, their, theirs
Positive-Sounding Words: and, additionally, we, us, our, together

Whilst it may be unnatural to substitute every single "negative" word with a "positive" word, in general speeches that contain the more positive-sounding words tend to be more inclusive and warmer, which means the audience prefer them, and hence the presentation succeeds more.

Thirdly, Do Not Overcomplicate: Virtually everybody sometimes overcomplicates an explanation at some time, but this is something presenters should actively try to avoid whilst presenting. It is good to aim for a style which appears professional but does not assume too much from the audience. Clearly, therefore, since audiences differ so much, the precise words to use will vary from occasion to occasion. The easiest trap to fall into is becoming too wordy. If you begin to sound verbose, that is a signal to simplify the explanation [2].

14.2.2 Body Language

There are three aspects of body language to consider:

First Aspect: Match the Body Language of Your Audience. Many different types of professionals will be familiar with the body language technique known as mirroring, which involves matching the posture, tone of voice, etc. of the person with whom you are communicating. Some readers may not be aware, however, that mirroring can also be applied when speaking on the telephone, in online meetings and at presentations. It is important to realise that mirroring works both ways. Thus, when you begin to mirror someone that person generally subconsciously begins to mirror you. This gives presenters an opportunity to mould the actions of the audience members. If some of your listeners seem to be distracted, for example, you can mirror them and then switch to a more attentive mode. This technique has been used with success to re-engage audience members in presentations.

Second Aspect: Become Very Comfortable with the Neutral Position. Adopting the neutral position is one of the most frequently given pieces of advice to presenters seeking to become more expert. In practice, however, this position is not as commonly adopted as might be expected. The advantages of the position are that it makes the presenter feel more comfortable as well as putting the audience at ease when they observe it. The following tips show how to assume the natural position.

- Keep your hands down by your sides. Do not place your hands in your pockets or cross them over your chest. You are not a shop window mannequin!
- Stand with a little more weight on one foot than the other. It is tiring to watch sometime standing like a guard on parade. Avoid shifting your weight from foot to foot or rocking.
- Allow your hand and arm gestures to flow naturally. There is no need to keep the elbows rigidly flexed. For online presentations, do not do anything which causes your webcam to shake, as this gives the audience motion sickness. Avoid grasp-

ing the monitor or shaking the camera, both of which appear very unprofessional when presenting [2].

Third Aspect: Record and Watch. Record yourself, watch your performance and think how to critique it. Repeat as many times as necessary. Some expert presenters do this as many as 20 times, but you may not need to aim for this level of perfectionism. In any case, every time you practise, your performance should steadily improve. Recording yourself, either in video or audio format, lets you see the presentation from the audience perspective, whether that is a C-suite meeting or a group of parents of school children. However, avoid simply memorising your lines. Ensure that you know the content very well, which then means you can present in a spontaneous and fluent manner. The only parts where memorisation is a bonus are if you think of an especially pithy concluding remark, witty aside or want to use particular phrases. The reason not to memorise the entire presentation is that merely reciting the lines will not make you seem fully engaged, and if this is so, your audience will not be fully engaged, either [2].

References

1. Using visual aids during a presentation or training session. https://virtualspeech.com/blog/visual-aids-presentation. Accessed 4 Oct 2021.
2. Marggraff B. The art of positive presentation. 4 Sept 2013. https://universityinnovationfellows.org/the-art-of-positive-presentation/. Accessed 4 Oct 2021.

15.1 Presenting Using Visuals

Visuals are an especially valuable way to reinforce the messages of any presentation. Despite their value, they are neglected by many presenters, who rely solely on the spoken or written word to put their message across. However, there are at least ten reasons why visual elements in presentations increase audience engagement and make the presentation much more memorable [1].

15.1.1 Use of Visuals Cuts Down on Preparation Time

To craft a compelling presentation often takes a high level of effort and investment of time. Much of this effort involves creating text. If appropriate visuals are chosen, the need for text is much lower and thus a considerable amount of time can be saved. Realistically, few audience members will have the inclination both to listen carefully to what the presenter says and to read the text on the slides. One or the other will inevitably not occur. However, it is reasonable to suppose an audience can look at visuals and listen to the presenter simultaneously.

15.1.2 Visuals Add Greater Interest to Presentations

Anyone who has listened to a number of presentations will have experienced being extremely bored by some presenters. Indeed, there is a sense in which PowerPoint now automatically evokes a tired reaction. To avoid this association of PowerPoint with lacklustre, text-heavy presentations, try using more photographic images and video clips to engage the audience. Skilfully employed visuals add fresh vigour and interest to a presentation.

C. C. Cingi et al., *Improving Online Presentations*,
https://doi.org/10.1007/978-3-031-28328-4_15

15.1.3 Visuals Are Effective at Creating Interest

In a nutshell, visuals are a key way to get your audience engaged. The audience members in any presentation frequently have difficulty grasping the main messages, particularly with complex or unfamiliar material. The Visual Teaching Alliance suggests that visuals are much more quickly understood than either text or spoken commentary. It takes no more than 0.1 s on average to comprehend what a visual represents, and in fact the processing of visual information occurs sixty thousand-fold higher than processing of written description. Presenters who omit visuals fail to utilise this major difference to their advantage.

15.1.4 Visuals Assist with Audience Comprehension

More than simply attracting the interest of an audience, the use of visuals assists with audience comprehension of information in a presentation. Forbes estimates that 65% of people have a primarily visual learning style. Bearing in mind that most speakers are aiming to create a strong image in the audience's mind, it seems more advantageous to present such an image directly, whenever possible. Indeed, some 90% of information flow in the brain is concerned with vision, so, utilising this modality is clearly sensible.

15.1.5 Visuals Make the Content of Presentations More Memorable

On average, people recall approximately 20% of spoken messages, but use of a visual stimulus increases retention four-fold. Researchers from Georgia State University have noted that visual imagery effectively improves memory. To increase how memorable your content is, intersperse text with appropriate visuals.

15.1.6 Visuals Improve the Efficiency of Communication

There are many people who lack the ability to speak in a truly effective way. The solution, however, is not, as might be imagined, a course in elocution, but rather to remember that the spoken aspect of your presentation is only one of the several communication channels that can be opened in a presentation. The visual channel is amongst the most important. By utilising high quality images, diagrams and video clips in a well-chosen way, the message can be enhanced and the presentation more effective at engaging the audience and conveying information to them.

15.1.7 Visuals May Create an Emotional Reaction

It is possible to describe an emotionally charged scene to someone and realise that, whilst they know what emotions to feel, they do not actually experience those emotions. To activate an audience's genuine and complete emotional response, it is better to let them witness the scene visually. Let them see what you mean. A skilled presenter can use images or video clips to get the audience to experience a range of emotions, from happiness and excitement through to sorrow or awe.

15.1.8 Effective Use of Visuals Promotes Inclusivity

It is a common mistake to consider audiences as possessing greater cognitive homogeneity than is really the case. An assumption of this kind fails to account for the linguistic, cultural and neuro-diversity found within groups. Since the audience will have varying abilities to grasp the meaning of a presentation, it is probable that some members of the audience will fail to grasp the entire meaning. By introducing visuals, you offer a different way for your audience to understand the meaning and thus include a greater number of people amongst those who fully understand the message.

15.1.9 Well-Chosen Visuals Enhance Audience Trust in the Message

If you want the audience to really trust you and your message, be sure to pick the highest quality images, well-produced videos and carefully designed infographics. If you produce your own content, this increases your own profile and credibility much more than relying on stock images or generic YouTube videos. A high degree of professionalism in choice and use of visuals will make your audience view you as highly professional and trustworthy.

15.1.10 Use Unique Visuals to Give Your Presentation Individuality

Utilising very common visual cliches is not the way to make your presentation stand out as different and unforgettable. Unique visuals, though, create the possibility of making your presentation truly outstanding. Photographic images and video footage that are created specifically for the presentation allow for a much greater degree of creative control than most presentations exhibit. Use visuals in a creative way that allows the maximum individuality to shine through.

15.2   Where Visuals Detract from Presentations

15.2.1 First Error: Visuals Used to Patch Problems

It is a big mistake to use visuals as a way to patch up a poor presenting technique, such as only including visuals to remind the presenter what to say, to fill in for insufficient content or to allow the presenter to try out a new laser pointer! This kind of misuse of visuals severely detracts from the effectiveness of those visuals that are genuinely appropriate and needed to convey your message.

15.2.2 Second Error: The Visuals Control You, Not the Other Way Round

Beware of letting your media control you, rather than the other way around. It is easy to feel that the more slides you have, the greater the impact, especially when the slides are visually appealing. But this is a mistake, since too many slides can easily turn excitement into boredom. There are various ways to decide how many slides is optimum. One common piece of advice is to have a fresh slide on average every minute. However, such rules of thumb are very rough guides. It is better to consider what number is most appropriate given your topic. If, for example, you need to present examples of where language errors happen, you might need a slower pace. A talk on work–life balance might not need any visuals at all. Where you do decide a visual would be appropriate, consider the purpose of showing the visual. Never just show slides to give the audience something to look at passively. The visuals are there to serve your objectives as a presenter, not as a separate, standalone component.

15.2.3 Third Error: Slides That Resemble a Shopping List

In terms of visual interest, the least effective slides are those consisting of full text. Excessive use of bullet point lists, however, comes in a close second. Too many lists resemble a shopping list, with items included to be comprehensive rather than comprehensible. Words are not inherently visual, even if the font is attractive and they are assembled nicely on a slide. Keep your words and visuals separate. True visuals consist of photographic images, infographics, original art, charts or cartoons. Of course, there may be a need to present text in a visually appealing manner, but in these cases, slides of this kind should not be seen as an alternative to a genuine visual. If a visual is needed, give the visual its own slide.

15.2.4 Fourth Error: Selecting the Wrong Visual

If you wish to illustrate how a machine or process works, suitable visuals are models, simulations or the actual machine. To show the inner mechanism of a device, photographs (enlarged if necessary), or line drawings, are appropriate. A trend can be easily made out on a line graph, which is clearer than a list of data points. Flow charts are good for illustrating an algorithm. Sales figures may be best shown on a bar chart and concepts may be illustrated through a cartoon or picture. Whatever message you want to convey, make sure that the visual is appropriate for that objective.

15.2.5 Fifth Mistake: Looking at the Visuals Rather Than the Audience

Visuals are shown to help the audience understand. They should already be familiar to the presenter, so face the audience, rather than your slide. Never read off from a slide. Aim to be sufficiently familiar with your content that you can present without turning away from the audience. Talk around the visual rather than just describing it.

15.2.6 Sixth Error: Letting the Slideshow Stop the Audience Seeing You

The presenter should be the focus of the audience's attention, rather than anything else. The audience come to hear a presenter, not read the slides. If you let the slides be the main focus, why not simply send the audience the slides and let them read them at home? If the slides are projected in such a way that you are forced into a corner of the stage, you will no longer be the focus of attention. In the majority of cases, a better solution is to have the screen at an angle, so that it does not cover the whole stage and the audience can see both the presenter and slideshow clearly.

15.2.7 Seventh Error: Presenting Messily

Presentations need to be concise and neatly expressed. If you include text, facts or visuals that do not reinforce your key message, your presentation will appear messy. Be careful not to add too much numerical information, as this can overwhelm an audience and obscure the message. Be concise. If you provide a handout that is the place to list any extra data needed to fully comprehend all the details. Use a limited number of font faces and point sizes. The font should not be distracting. Choose a font on the basis of maximum legibility. Leave plenty of clear space on slides so that people viewing the slide can easily take in the whole slide. If animations are to be used, ensure that they reinforce the message and do not confuse the audience with irrelevancies, such as swirling banners, flashing lights and extra sound effects.

15.2.8 Eighth Error: Overloading Slides

Each slide should convey just one key idea. The use of visuals is justified by the need to clarify a concept. If the visual ends up requiring its own lengthy explanation, it would be better omitted.

15.2.9 Ninth Error: Overcomplicated Slide Transitions and Build Slides

The use of slide transitions and build slides has a drastic effect on the speed of the presentation. Some types of transition really slow the pace, and some build effects can be distracting, if text comes flying in from all directions at once.

A build slide may make a subject easier to present and easier to take in for the audience but will be slower to present than a conventional static slide. If the entire text is present from the start, it is easier to abbreviate the presentation when you are running behind time. You can explain that you are omitting particular sections rather than just not mentioning them at all. Interested members of the audience can quickly read through the full list and follow up later. It is important therefore to consider all the possible scenarios when presenting, both when everything goes according to plan and when things go wrong, such as when you are short of time [2].

15.3   Visuals

Visuals that are effective in a presentation are [3]

- Of sufficient size
- In the correct format
- Memorable
- Fit the content of the other slides
- Trigger the desired emotional response

Having considered both effective and ineffective uses of visuals, we can now consider seven sources of visuals that are suited to use in presentations.

15.3.1 Utilise Stock Photos in Preparing Presentations

Many people are wary of using stock photos as visuals. However, whereas there are some stock photos which give a cliched look to a presentation (think "impossibly perfect family smiling cheesily"), if a high quality stock photo supplies your requirements, there is no need to avoid using it. Be selective.

15.3.2 Make Use of Icons

Icons are a quick and straightforward way to add visual interest to a slide.

There are some websites that offer downloadable icons. Some are also included in certain software packages, such as PowerPoint or LibreOffice.

There are hundreds of icons, and these are well-constructed from a graphical point of view. Use high quality icons rather than ones which resemble poor quality clip-art.

The icons included within PowerPoint fulfil these requirements well. They are clean-looking, elegant and contemporary.

Icons can be used within infographics or charts, where they add visual interest and improve comprehensibility [3].

15.3.3 Use Photos You Have Taken Yourself

Many presenters consider the use of stock photographic images, but it is unusual to see presenters use their own photos. However, this is a resource that definitely should not be overlooked, since your own photos are both original and royalty-free.

15.3.4 Produce Your Own Artwork to Accompany Slides

Yes, you read that correctly. You can produce your own artwork for presentations.

Many people instinctively feel that their own artwork would be unsuitable for a presentation; however, it is worth bearing the following in mind:

- Hand drawings are much more eye-catching and appealing than most types or stock footage or generic visual.
- Audiences tend to remember hand drawings much more easily and these drawings are very helpful for increasing audience understanding.

Even if you may not be a particularly talented artist, it is more important to interest and engage your audience than to bore them with dull, professional images [3].

15.3.5 Some Animated Gifs Add Emotional Relief

Animated gifs can make your audience smile or laugh and are a very effective way to give some relief to the mood in a serious presentation. Make your audience see the humorous side once in a whilst to maintain engagement. Audiences will realise you can empathise with them [3].

15.3.6 Make Use of Internet Memes

The way to use memes is similar to animated gifs. They help lighten a mood and establish a connection with the audience.

Memes are easy to search for online. They can be freely reproduced, since they lack the copyright restrictions which exist on most images you can find online.

Because memes are very specific, it is usually straightforward to find the exact meme you want to use [3].

15.3.7 Make Use of Video Clips

The last option is to show video clips in your presentation.

The types of video suitable include:

- Videos on the internet (from sites like YouTube or Dailymotion)
- Video in DVD or other standard video format

It is generally better to avoid the use of video clips which are already hosted online, for several reasons. In particular, when you link to a video hosted online:

- The presentation has a tendency to lose momentum.
- Showing a video like this may make your internet connection become unstable in a Zoom session.
- You are at the mercy of internet outages.

Whilst it is often possible to download a copy of such videos for offline use, it may be unethical to do so. For one thing, content creators are typically paid for views and receive no recompense when you view offline.

Therefore, where there is definite value in getting the audience to view a particular video clip, it may be better to send the link prior to, or following, the presentation, instead [3].

15.4   Use of Positives

A straightforward, yet effective technique to increase the impact from a presentation is to introduce "positives" (i.e. words with a positive connotation) into your delivery. The use of positives tends to improve the audience's mood. Some presenters refer to such words as "power words". This technique should be applied sparingly, to avoid ruining the effect [4].

Positive words to use in the introduction
1. Thanks, e.g. "Many thanks for this opportunity to speak to you".
2. Lovely. "It is lovely to be here once more".
3. Nice. "It is really nice to see so many familiar faces".
4. Passionate. "This is a topic we are all so passionate about".

Positive words for learning and discovering
5. Show. "This presentation will show what it is all about".
6. Learn. "You have an opportunity to learn…"
7. Find. "Finding the meaning…"
8. Discover. "Discovery brings its own thrill".
9. New. "This is the new reality".
10. Found. "Researchers found something unexpected…"

Positive words regarding content
11. Clearly. "These results clearly reveal…"
12. Impressive. "What could be more impressive?"
13. Very. "They were very committed to doing it".
14. Positive. "A really positive advance".
15. Lot. "This answers a lot of questions".
16. Importance. "The result is of great importance to all of us".
17. Cool. "Not only surprising, but also very cool".
18. Great. "A great outcome".
19. Good. "A good compromise".
20. Marvellous. "Marvellous work".
21. Wonderful. "The wonderful men and women who work in…"
22. Totally. "Totally reliable" [4].

Positive words to use when ending a presentation
23. Enjoyment. "Speaking has brought me a great deal of enjoyment".
24. Pleasure. "It was a real pleasure to hear your questions".
25. Thank you. "Thank you very much indeed for your time".

References

1. 10 reasons why you need good presentation visuals. 13 June 2021. https://www.splento.com/blog/photography/10-reasons-why-you-need-good-presentation-visuals/. Accessed 4 Oct 2021.

2. Booher D. 9 mistakes presenters make with visuals. https://www.ou.edu/class/prestech/articles/9%20Mistakes%20Presenters%20Make%20with%20Visuals.htm. Accessed 4 Oct 2021.
3. How to make visual presentations: 7 types of visuals you can use in your presentation slides right now. https://www.echorivera.com/blog/7visuals. Accessed 4 Oct 2021.
4. The Top 25 Positive Words to use in your Presentation. https://www.presentationmagazine.com/top-positive-words-presentation-16762.htm. Accessed 4 Oct 2021.

16.1 Presenting Positively

Many people have a fear of delivering presentations, but in contemporary professional life, the presentation plays a key role. The fear that accompanies public speaking is hard to completely conquer, but would-be presenters can learn techniques to manage their anxiety. Furthermore, presenting successfully on one occasion is very effective at reducing the anxiety of presenting on future occasions. Success really does breed success.

So, for anyone faced with the prospect of delivering a presentation soon, it is important to be able to identify those aspects of delivery which mark the difference between success and failure. The following are key points to consider [1].

16.1.1 Confidence

Whilst it may be hard to sound genuinely confident, appearing confident is a surefire way of making your audience engaged and convinced. The audience then want your presentation to be successful and want you to give them confidence, too. Presenters who are unsure of how to deliver a presentation and who stumble over their words are not likely to sell their ideas or products to an audience. However, if presenters have prepared themselves adequately, this comes across as appropriate confidence, and their performance is likely to be excellent [1].

16.1.2 Passion

Maintaining a high level of audience engagement in a presentation is far from simple, particularly in business contexts. Although presentations usually cover important subjects, there is a tendency for content to be fairly indigestible. The presenter needs to transform the subject into something lively and interesting. Audiences watching an enthusiastic presenter frequently go on to develop their own enthusiasm for the topic. Thus, if you speak with genuine passion and eloquence, as a minimum you keep your listeners focused on the presentation, and with luck you inspire them with enthusiasm for the subject [1].

16.1.3 Knowledge

Prior to putting together a presentation, research your topic in depth and ensure you are as knowledgeable as possible about the subject. Ideally, you should be at the level where you can confidently discuss the topic in detail without any notes or slides to fall back on. Unless you acquire some level of expertise on the subject you are presenting, the audience will sense that you are simply parroting a few facts and will rapidly lose their confidence in you and become bored by the presentation [1].

16.1.4 Being Yourself

Even though presenters may feel more confident in presenting if they have memorised what they want to say, delivery of a memorised speech often leaves an audience dissatisfied. Whilst professionalism is an essential component, there needs also to be a human touch. If you know your topic really well, you can present in a more natural and spontaneous fashion, and this style always promotes better audience engagement. By all means ensure you cover the main material and do not deviate into irrelevancies, but allow a certain amount of room for manoeuvre, to make the whole presentation more enjoyable and relaxed.

16.1.5 Organisation

Spontaneous, natural delivery is important for presenters, but the presentation itself should be very well-organised and adhere to a proper structure. Presenters who skip from subject to subject are apt to confuse the audience, even if they do manage to cover all the material. The topics need to follow on from each other in a logical, coherent manner. A properly organised presentation is much more straightforward for an audience to follow and thus more likely to succeed in delivering its key messages [1].

16.1.6 Timekeeping

The requirement to be comprehensive in your treatment of a topic must be balanced against the need to avoid the presentation becoming excessively long. Whatever the topic, if the presentation lasts too long, your audience will stop attending to what you are saying. Aim for a concise treatment. If you need to, do not be afraid to omit material, only retaining what is absolutely essential. When you actually deliver the presentation, be prepared to further reduce the material presented if there is a danger of over-running [1].

16.1.7 Be Clear

The central objective of all presentations is successful communication of a message. Even if the presentation has all the features described above, without the audience grasping the central message, the presentation as a whole must be considered a failure. You should be very confident that you know what message you want to give and should ensure that is the actual message you send. Keep the central message in mind throughout the presentation. Being clear about the message to deliver is the key to achieving clarity in the presentation as a whole and being successful presenting [1].

16.2   How to Deliver a Presentation Well

An effective presentation begins with well-chosen content. Your message may be extremely important, but unless you can reduce the subject to a comprehensible set of slides and accompanying narration, you have no way of convincing an audience. The following sections outline how to create and organise your content [2].

16.2.1 Structure the Material so that the Audience Can Easily Follow

In virtually every presentation, the content should be arranged around a three-section structure consisting of introduction, body and conclusion.

- **A powerful introduction** gives the audience advanced notice of the material to follow and sets it into context. It explains why the audience will benefit from hearing the presentation.
- **Supply Supporting Evidence for Your Argument in the Body:** This is where the key evidence to support your argument is assembled and presented. Evidence includes data, quotations, case studies, etc.
- **Conclude by Reiterating the Important Points:** In the final section, you restate your argument, reiterate the main message and let the audience now what you expect them to take away from the presentation, whether that is particular knowledge or an action you want them to perform.
- **Ten Slides Are Usually Sufficient:** For short presentations, the number of slides should not normally exceed ten. More than that number tends to mean the audience lose focus. Even if the presentation lasts half an hour, using fewer slides

means the audience can comfortably keep up with the key messages. To ensure that the slides perform their function of reinforcing the central message, many experts recommend the use of concept maps [2] when putting together a slide set.

16.2.2 Do Not Overcrowd the Slides

Slides are always more effective when they do not contain too much information. If a slide is too crowded, the audience tend to concentrate on the slide rather than listening to your narration. Not only do they become distracted, they may also miss the key clues in your tone of voice, body language and other aspects of delivery.

- **Slides May Contain as few as Six Words:** Some experts, such as the marketing guru Seth Godin, take the approach of minimal text to an extreme. He recommends no more than six words per slide, in an attempt to maintain maximum focus.
- **Information Should Be Bite-Sized:** Audiences should not feel they have bitten off more than they can chew. Keep the amount of information at a level where no one feels over-faced. Other formats also help make information more digestible. Video is said to be 95% more convincing as a medium than simple text [2].

16.2.3 Know the Principles of Good Design

The difference between success and failure sometimes comes down to how well-designed the presentation is. Although hiring a professional to design your slides may be ideal, for many people a more economical approach is to use a service like Visme or Canva, with images chosen from the royalty-free collections on Pexels or Unsplash.

- **Use a Restricted Palate:** Although being colourful is generally an attractive feature, avoid using too many separate colours. It is best to keep to a few colours (up to four, including black and white) if you want to give the same "look-and-feel" to the entire presentation.
- **Text Should Have a Consistent Appearance:** Switching frequently between fonts gives an amateurish impression. Likewise, avoid excessive alteration of ALL CAPITALS and all lower case. Keep to one font and one point size for most of the presentation. Do not mix fonts. If you want to emphasise a particular word, it is better to indicate this by altering your tone of voice when you present rather than by altering the appearance of certain words. A consistent text is easier to read.
- **Avoid Formatting Errors:** Errors such as a low resolution image at large size or a misplaced line are distracting and may make the presenter appear careless about details. Ensure that the text lines up, and that everything has a neat appearance when projected [2].

16.2.4 Repeated Polishing Pays Off

As with anything else you want to put on public display, polishing your presentation repeatedly will create a more positive impression.

- **Do Not Worry About Neatness to Begin With:** There are tools, such as Milanote, that let presenters sketch out their ideas before trying to generate slides in PowerPoint or other presentation software. When you give yourself the freedom to experiment in this way, you may uncover unexpected connections between topics and increase your own understanding.
- **Keep Pruning:** The initial drafts will probably contain much more material than you can comfortably present. This is where it pays to prune the material until only the absolutely essential content needed to support your message is left.

Have a colleague or friend review your slides first. Getting an objective opinion from someone else, whose opinion you can trust, is very valuable for finding mistakes and areas requiring improvement. If there is nobody who can perform such a role for you, you may find that software grammar checkers, such as ProWritingAid or Grammarly are helpful in identifying errors in how you express yourself.

The way you actually deliver your presentation is as significant as the content and appearance of your slides. The following advice will assist in delivering your message with maximum effectiveness [2].

16.2.5 Create a Powerful Beginning

Strong introductory and concluding sections of a presentation are especially vital to the success of any presentation. In most cases, the audience form their initial impression about the presenter and the presentation within the first 5–10 s. Getting the beginning right is therefore essential if you are to succeed.

- **Be Original:** Find an original angle on your material that will make your audience laugh or smile. For example, if you are presenting about a new type of laptop, you could tell the audience a tale about the time your young daughter thought your notebook was a real book and drew all over the cover in brightly coloured crayons. Audiences will relate to the story and start to engage with you and the material.
- **Pose Questions:** Rhetorical questions are a way to get the audience to think or feel certain ideas. Imagine that you are presenting new social legislation designed to protect vulnerable children. Try asking, "How many children had to die for the law to finally change?"
- **Fit Your Approach to the Audience:** The more presenters understand their audience, the greater their chance of really succeeding. In particular, make sure you know their preferences and priorities. Include references that they can

identify with. Barack Obama, when visiting Jamaica, was able to say a few sentences in Jamaican patois, which won his audience over immediately [2].

16.2.6 Be True to Yourself

As Shakespeare said in Hamlet (Act 1, Scene 3):

> *This above all: to thine own self be true,*
> *And it must follow, as the night the day,*
> *Thou canst not then be false to any man.*

For any subject, speak about the subject in the way you feel most comfortable. Do not see the presentation as an opportunity to prove yourself. Concentrate instead on getting the message across in the way you want. The whole point of any presentation is to deliver certain messages. If you succeed in conveying those messages, your job as a presenter is complete.

- **Employ Your Sense of Humour:** Humour adds a great deal to effective delivery, but do not try too hard to be witty. An amusing story helps make you and your message easier to relate to and people remember it for longer. In most presentations, people are happy to laugh at such stories. However, do not push too hard if the story falls flat, as it will destroy the audience's enjoyment.
- **Conquer Any Fear of Failure**: Many people become highly anxious when faced with presenting, as they fear failing in front of many people. It is better not to worry too much about such an occurrence. After all, nearly all actors or comedians have "died on stage" at some point in their careers. The UK magician, Paul Daniels, turned a heckler's remark into his signature catchphrase: "You'll like it...not a lot!"
- **Be Open and Reveal Your Vulnerability:** The fact that public speaking is a nerve-wracking experience for many people is not lost on the audience, who can often empathise with your feelings and admire your courage in speaking. If you are prepared to expose yourself a little to criticism, you will be very likely to win over the audience [2]. Tell your story, even if it is not easy to tell.

16.2.7 Planning for a Faultless Delivery

Since there is so much involved in deciding on what material to include and how to design your slides or visuals, you could be forgiven for overlooking the need to plan delivery in such a way as to minimise potential hitches. But this would be a mistake. There are in fact a number of ways to plan for a faultless delivery.

- **Practise Your Delivery, Ideally on Camera:** As a minimum, you should go through the delivery at least once before the actual presentation event. If it is possible, make a video recording, so that you can ensure you spot any potential problems in timing, flow and the manner in which you express yourself.

- **Utilise a Remote Control to Advance Slides:** A device of this sort gives the presenter much-needed freedom of movement. Presenters can continue to face the audience throughout the presentation, with no need to keep returning to their laptops. This allows for a more natural and flowing presentation style.
- **Prepare Backup Content:** Sometimes you may feel that the material you are presenting is not convincing your audience. In this situation, you need backup content, so that you can approach the topic from a different angle. There is also always a real possibility of equipment failure. If this occurs, expert speakers usually have some anecdotes at the ready that they can recount to fill in the missing content and to keep the audience engaged whilst the problem is being rectified. Having backup of this sort helps a presenter feel ready for any eventuality.
- **Stick Strictly to Time. Use a Stopwatch:** During delivery of a presentation, presenters can easily deviate from the main topic, especially in response to audience questions. Timing suffers as a result. It is good practice to set a stopwatch (often on a smartphone) to allow you to check your own timing as you go along [2].

16.2.8 The Key to Success Is Focusing on Value for the Audience

As you approach the final section of your presentation, how can you make sure the audience finds your message deeply memorable? Presentation experts agree that the key to this is deciding what emotions you want the audience to leave with.

- **Let the Last Message Be Emotional in Character:** Whilst it is easy to forget the words someone uses, if a person's words evoke a strong emotional response in you, that emotion will remain fixed in your memory. Give your last section an emotional tone by including a song, a line of poetry or anything else which will resonate strongly with your audience's emotions.
- **Remember the Value of Silence:** Silences are powerful. Leave a silence after any point that you especially want to emphasise. The silence helps the audience to focus on the message and derive greater meaning from it.
- **Let the Central Message Stand Out Clearly:** If you want to end your presentation in a strong way, challenge your audience to act on the consequences of your central message. Tell the audience what action they can undertake. Some presenters tell one final story, with an emphasis on emotion, to illustrate how this call to action can be answered [2].

References

1. 7 qualities of a good presentation. https://www.boomersplus.com/7-qualities-of-a-good-presentation/. Accessed 4 Oct 2021.
2. How to make a good presentation with 8 pro tips. https://biteable.com/blog/how-to-make-good-presentation/. Accessed 4 Oct 2021.

Visual Perception and Impairment. Presenting for Every Audience

17

17.1 Visual Perception and Awareness

People's perception of the world is enormously influenced by the things we see all around, including in the media. The eyes act as our guides, to show us which direction to take. Much of our reasoning depends on what our eyes perceive and the way in which they do so. If we are able to distinguish between objective appearance and our subjective visual perceptions, our visual awareness will grow. In physiological terms, vision depends on light rays entering the eye and being focused by the lens onto the retina. The retina is covered with light-sensitive cells which convert the light into electrical signals in the nervous system. The brain reassembles these electrical signals to form the image that we are subjectively aware of. Modern life presents us with so rich a visual environment, particularly through media, that much of what we perceive is not specifically attended to by our minds. A lot of what we see carries no particular meaning. Visual awareness is more than just this relatively passive act of perceiving images, since other factors play a role in how we generate visual meaning. For example, our previous experience, pre-formed ideas, wishes and concepts all affect what we perceive as the "evident truth". Culture also modulates how we perceive the world. Think of the difference between an arm raised by a traffic policeman to signal the need to stop before an accident occurs and the same gesture performed by a far right extremist [1].

To put it slightly differently, we can note that "seeing" and "looking" are not synonymous. Looking involves glancing in a particular direction and being aware of when something enters our gaze. Seeing is a more complex process that involves understanding. This is the reason why "I see" is synonymous with "I understand". Seeing involves attaching meaning to what we perceive visually. Faced with the vast volume of visual information that modern lifestyles throw at us, we need to decide what to genuinely see, rather than just notice. People concentrate on seeing whatever holds most significance for them, such as a motorway sign indicating the turning they need to take or a beautiful view from a hotel window. When information is

C. C. Cingi et al., *Improving Online Presentations*, https://doi.org/10.1007/978-3-031-28328-4_17

delivered via our screens, we see what attracts us, whether that is the weather forecast or an important e-mail we are expecting. By focusing our visual perception, we begin to see and therefore understand. Furthermore, the act of attending visually to a stimulus, such as a painting or a panoramic view, leads us to form an aesthetic perception. We judge its beauty or attractiveness. This aesthetic judgement considers just the visual qualities of the object, comparing them with our previous aesthetic preferences. The judgement helps us to deduce the meaning of our visual perception [1].

Nonetheless, visual perceptions, however acute, are insufficient to generate a really deep understanding of a subject. What is needed is language, which may be in the form of a written text accompanying the image or a spoken commentary. Words supply the context for the aesthetic perception. If we know the historical background, the religious meaning or the cultural function of an object, we can appreciate its value as a work of art. This is the reason why galleries or museums offer guides and written information about the items on display and why people consult experts on art. This extra information contextualises the object and lets us understand (see) its true meaning [1].

17.2 Increasing the Accessibility of a Visually Based Presentation

When a presentation is to be delivered, you, the presenter, need to consider carefully how to maximise audience accessibility to the presentation and your commentary. Visual impairments are very common and indeed, on a global scale some 314 million people suffer from a visual disability, the WHO estimates. Dyslexia is also common, possibly affecting 4% of people. Thus, the likelihood of an audience member having such a barrier to accessibility is relatively high [2].

17.2.1 Design Considerations for Presentations

In the next few sections we will look at some suggestions for preparing slides using presentation software. PowerPoint is the most common software used for this purpose, but there are alternatives, such as writing the presentation in HTML. A poster may also be suitable. However you decide to present, the following suggestions are all designed to increase accessibility [2].

17.2.2 Size and Volume of Text on Individual Slides

- There should be no more than six lines of text, with each line containing a maximum of six words.
- Align the text to the left margin.

- The size of text is chosen so that a person with a degree of visual impairment sitting at the front would find it legible, as would a person without visual impairment sitting on the back row. This means in general that **text is at least 32 points**.
- Use sentence case in preference to all capitals [2].

17.2.3 Font Face

- Fonts lacking serifs project best. Helvetica, Arial or Verdana are all suitable.
- Do not use italics.
- Ideally, a slide should not utilise more than a single font [2].

17.2.4 Achieve Contrast with Different Colours and Degree of Brightness

- To make a slide easier for visually impaired people to see, create a colour contrast between the background and foreground.
- Contrast can be achieved using colour or brightness.
- Brightness contrast is maximal between black and white.
- To achieve maximum colour contrast, use complementary colours.
- If the contrast is based on colour alone, particularly red contrasted with green, this may present difficulties for people with colour blindness. Therefore, brightness levels should also be contrasted.
- Since glare may create difficulty, light text on a dark background is safer than vice versa. White text written on dark blue background is especially legible [2].

17.2.5 Figures and Graphs

- Simplify figures or graphs wherever possible.
- Apply the same principles about contrast achieved with colour or brightness levels to graphs and figures as to text.
- For text in figures, use a font lacking serifs [2].

17.2.6 Animations

- Only use animation where absolutely essential [2].

17.2.7 Provide a Verbal Description of the Slides

- During your introduction, outline what format the presentation will follow and when questions may be asked.

- Read any text that is written on the slides.
- Talk through any figures or graphs.
- Rather than merely pointing to the key area on a slide, explain in words.
- Express clearly to the audience which parts of a slide you are presenting.
- Where a slide is text-heavy, go through it at a moderate pace and with maximum verbal clarity [2].

17.2.8 Handouts

- Prior to starting delivery, give out handouts containing the information on the slides.
- Colour contrast is lost if the handouts are black and white.
- Keep some full page printouts of the slides for those audience members who have visual problems [2].

17.2.9 Assisting Blind Audience Members

- Keep copies of the presentation on a USB flash disc, for easy transfer to a blind person's laptop. It is even better if you can supply a Braille handout. A CD is a further alternative you could offer.
- A copy of the presentation may be posted to an internet site in html format, with a downloadable .pdf or .pps version.
- Whatever you show needs to have an audio description. One way to ensure this is to think how you would adapt your presentation to deliver it on the radio or as a podcast [2].

17.3 Best Practices for Online Delivery

Since the COVID-19 pandemic began, presenting online has become a routine part of life for many people. Whilst many of the techniques needed for effective delivery face-to-face are similar to those used online, there are differences which virtual presenters need to be familiar with if they wish to fully succeed. In a face-to-face presentation, you already have considerable buy-in from your audience before you begin, and it is unusual for audience members to leave part way through. This is not the case with online presentations, where presenters are competing for the attention of their audiences against distractions in the home or office, other demands on the audience members' time and a generally lower ability to focus on a single topic [3].

The following advice is intended to improve your chances of a successful online presentation [3].

17.3.1 Ensure Adequate Illumination

The presenter needs to be clearly visible during a presentation. Light should fall from the front, not the back, as this casts you into shadow. If you present with a window behind you, it may be necessary to close the blind or curtains. The highest quality illumination comes from natural light, but if you frequently appear online from an office without natural light, separate special lighting may be better than relying on the room's overhead lights, as it will offer a more flattering light source [3].

17.3.2 Select an Appropriate Background

The background against which you present sends a message about your professionalism. It should also reflect the message of your presentation. Aim for an uncluttered background free of distractions. Some videoconferencing solutions, such as Zoom or Microsoft Teams, allow use of a virtual background (an image that appears to be behind the presenter). It is also possible to blur the actual background to prevent it being clearly seen. A suitable background reinforces a professional image, whereas an unsuitable one tends to appear amateurish at best [3].

17.3.3 Familiarise Yourself with the Software and Equipment First

Presenters who appear unable to use the presentation equipment and software destroy the audience's confidence in the presentation. Presenting is a performance, for which rehearsal is essential. Having a co-presenter or moderator to help with the housekeeping activities is beneficial in terms of letting a presenter focus on the presentation. It also means someone else can help in case of technical issues. For a rehearsal to be most useful to you, you need to practise with the same software and equipment that you will be using on the day of the actual presentation [3].

17.3.4 Address the Camera

Whilst speaking, look at the webcam or other camera, rather than at the screen, where you can see the audience. Although this feels rather unintuitive, the effect for the audience is that you are making eye contact. It may be helpful to turn off the view of yourself since this can be misleading. The camera should be placed at the level of your eyes. Below this level, the angle tends to emphasise your chin, whereas above this level you may appear to keep looking down as it is tiring to keep your head turned upwards all the time. Be careful about knowing when the camera is on. It is easy to be caught off guard doing something embarrassing, like yawning or scratching. Whilst another speaker is presenting, be sure to appear attentive. Just as with any presentation, eye contact makes a huge difference, so be prepared to set up the camera to imitate this action [3].

17.3.5 Stand Near Enough to the Camera

Ideally, your face, neck and shoulders should be caught on camera. If your face is clearly visible, that helps an audience to feel connected to you, however it is important that your face does not fill the entire screen as this is disconcertingly close for an audience. Experiment until you find the optimal distance away from the camera [3].

17.3.6 Stand in Preference to Sitting

Whenever feasible, it is better to stand when presenting, with the camera at eye level. To achieve this a standing desk may help. When we stand, our voice contains more energy and the rest of the body is in a more natural position to deliver a presentation. If standing is not an option, be sure to lean towards the camera, which conveys interest and engagement. In fact, this is the posture generally adopted by TV newsreaders or people sitting in a face-to-face meeting and is far preferable to leaning backwards, which gives an arrogant or uninterested air [3].

17.3.7 Be Energetic

In virtual presentations, just like in face-to-face events, being energetic is an advantage. If the pace is too slow or your voice remains monotonous, the audience can easily give up and leave the presentation. Virtual audiences only become engaged in a presentation in response to an active effort by the presenter [3].

17.3.8 Keep an Eye on Your Speed

Pacing yourself online is more challenging than face-to-face, since there are fewer clues coming from the audience about how they are reacting. Although presentations should be energetic and lively, avoid getting faster and faster. Consider your normal speed of speaking—if you tend to speak very quickly, adjust the pace down a little. Conversely, slow speakers may need to up the pace somewhat to maintain momentum [3].

17.3.9 Check How Clear Your Voice Is

The audience tend not to pay attention if your voice signal is unclear. Online audiences are more tolerant of a poor video signal than a poor audio signal. The latter is a frequent reason for exiting a presentation. It is worth checking how clear your voice sounds by getting a friend to connect remotely. If the audio signal is unclear, it may be worth seeing whether using the computer's own microphone or an external microphone or headset is better. There are a number of factors that operate to produce a clear sound signal, so experiment a little, then use the best combination of equipment when you present [3].

17.3.10   Ethernet Is More Stable than Wireless

Where possible, use a wired connection (such as Ethernet) rather than wireless since it provides a more reliable connection. Do whatever you can to prevent an unstable internet connection ruining your otherwise excellent presentation [3].

17.3.11   Arrange a Backup in Case of Technical Failure

If you have slides to present, leave a copy with the session moderator, so that, if the worst comes to the worst and you cannot open the slide set, he or she can do so on your behalf. Slides should be pleasant to look at. Any graphics need to be of high quality. Avoid overloading slides with text. The presenter's task, after all, is to deliver the message of the presentation and the slides are just there to complement what the presenter is saying [3]. Too much text on the slides means the audience will just focus on reading the slides instead.

17.3.12   Aim for Maximum Audience Engagement

Engaging your audience is just as important online as it is face-to-face, if not more so. Get the audience involved by allowing chats, doing polls and asking for audience reactions (thumbs up, yes/no, etc.). Aim to interact with your audience at least once every 10 min. Use the names of your audience, which should appear in the list of participants. If someone wants to ask a question or make a comment, let them do so by writing it in the chat box or using the "raise hand" feature. If there are multiple questions or comments, take them in order. You can ask them to unmute themselves to speak. They may also wish to turn on their camera [3].

17.3.13 Appoint Someone to Monitor the Chat on Your Behalf

Avoid being distracted by reading the chat messages as you present. It is easy to underestimate the difficulty of concentrating on both the chat and your delivery simultaneously. If you ask the audience a question or request feedback, remember to pause the presenting to thank the audience for their input and to read out all or some of the responses [3].

17.3.14 Assess your Own Performance and Aim to Improve

Whenever possible, record any presentations that you deliver so that you can watch it again afterwards and identify where you want to improve. Presenters who excel do so by constantly critiquing and improving on their own performance. However, when you critique your own performance, remember to focus on both positive and negative aspects. If some aspect went particularly well, remember how you did it, for subsequent re-use [3].

17.3.15 Be Genuine and Enjoy Presenting

Both in online and in face-to-face presentations, audiences are most drawn to presenters who seem genuine. Allow yourself to act naturally. Try to enjoy the opportunity to present and let the audience see you are happy. It has been established by researchers that a happy mood is associated with greater retention of information from a presentation. When the audience see you smiling and enthusiastic, they tend to mirror your mood and listen more attentively.

Above all, any presentation, whatever the format, is a performance event. The whole point of the presentation is to give value to the audience. Time is precious for everyone, and expert presenters give the maximum value to audiences in that time. Furthermore, regardless of the content you present, the way to put your message across always boils down to engaging the audience, creating genuine interest and giving them something of value through the way you deliver [3].

References

1. M1-ideas of perception and visual awareness. https://learn.canvas.net/courses/24/pages/m1-ideas-of-perception-and-visual-awareness. Accessed 4 Oct 2021.
2. How to make visual presentations accessible to audience members with print impairments. World Blind Union. https://2018.ifla.org/wp-content/uploads/2018/02/wbu-visual-presentations-guidelines-summary.pdf. Accessed 4 Oct 2021.
3. Abbajay M. Best practices for virtual presentations: 15 expert tips that work for everyone. 2020. https://www.forbes.com/sites/maryabbajay/2020/04/20/best-practices-for-virtual-presentations-15-expert-tips-that-work-for-everyone/?sh=170b9903d196. Accessed 4 Oct 2021.

Effective Endings: Leaving the Audience Impressed and Informed

18.1 Ending Your Presentation

Research findings indicate that individuals who attempt to recall information they were told earlier only really recall the beginning and end of the information. Thus, if you want the audience to go away with the right message from your presentation, a powerful concluding section is essential. If the ending does not fill your audience with inspiration and enthusiasm, they will most likely rapidly forget the message. Conversely, a powerful ending motivates the audience to action and fills them with the strength to act [1].

So, what are the best ways to ensure an effective ending? The following are some of the necessary techniques and points to bear in mind [1]:

18.1.1 Keep to the Time Limit

Although it might appear self-evident that good timekeeping is essential, a surprisingly large number of presenters do actually over-run their allocated time slot. This often results from presenters trying too hard to fill in every detail in the presentation, causing them to hurry and go beyond the normal finishing time.

Keeping to your time slot is a way of showing respect towards your busy audience. It makes you appear well-organised and someone who plans effectively. In other words, you appear the type of person worth listening to and following his or her advice.

18.1.1.1 Timekeeping Tactics

Do not forget to account for the time needed for audience questions and comments at the end. This time is valuable for increasing interactivity in the presentation.

Make it clear from the start of the presentation that you aim to stick to time and get your audience to co-operate in achieving this objective by saving questions for

C. C. Cingi et al., *Improving Online Presentations*, https://doi.org/10.1007/978-3-031-28328-4_18

later and not allowing themselves to be distracted by interesting off-topic questions and comments.

As your presentation concludes and is within the time limit, ensure that you remind the audience of your promise to finish in a timely way and express gratitude for their assistance in making this happen [1].

18.1.2 Make It Clear When You Have Finished Presenting

With some presenters, the presentation seems to just peter out, with a tendency for the audience to start talking to each other or, even more unsatisfactorily, with an agonising silence. This is a situation to avoid. Instead, let the audience clearly know that you have finished presenting, perhaps by thanking them for listening, saying goodbye or waving as you leave the stage. However you choose to do it, make it clear that the presentation is now over and the audience can safely leave [1].

18.1.3 End by Telling a Story

Telling a story is a very powerful way of affecting an audience during a presentation. However, many presenters fail to capitalise on this technique. There is a considerable literature concerning the value gained from storytelling in general, but suffice it to say that a well-told story has the ability to engage your audience, including on an emotional level, and to strengthen the key message. People will remember the story later, too.

A story should not be too lengthy for the ending section. Keep it short and personally relevant, by saying something like: "Just before we finish, I would like to tell you about something that happened to me recently…" [1].

18.1.4 Complete the Circle to Round Off Your Presentation

Let the audience feel the circle has been completed by referring at the end to the way you started your presentation. This gives a feeling of satisfying completion and makes the whole presentation seem unified.

Completing the circle in this way calls for a certain degree of planning. There are various ways to close the circle, such as:

- By asking a question at the start and providing an answer in the conclusion.
- Beginning a story at the start, with the ending provided as you draw the presentation to a close.
- Showing your first slide again at the end. This technique is especially effective if the slide has strong visual appeal or contains a memorable quote.
- Relate the presentation to a comment made by a member of the audience during an interactive activity at the start of the presentation.

18.1.5 Close with Your Opening Title

Sometimes, the presenter may wish to use the opening title as a way to end the presentation. This "title close" method has the advantage that it really emphasises what the central subject of the presentation is and how your message relates to the content.

Using the title close technique is analogous to the back cover of a printed book. It helps to set limits to the presentation as a whole.

18.1.6 Always Remain Upbeat and Enthusiastic

A presentation offers a magnificent opportunity to motivate, inspire and enthuse an audience. Some subjects naturally tend to be upbeat, but even where this is not the case and there are negative aspects to what you present, always make sure you leave room for hope.

Virtually any presentation can become inspiring if the presenter wishes it to be so. Indeed, the opportunity to inspire should never be neglected. You can inspire your audience in multiple ways, as follows:

- Employ lively, colourful and imaginative language
- Align the message with your audience's long term goals
- Keep long term goals in sight, not immediate agreement
- Above all, display optimism, positivity and energy [1]

18.1.7 Sound Bites

Sound bites resemble slogans or catch phrases in being very catchy and memorable. To create a sound bite, you need to condense the entire message of your presentation into a short, highly meaningful phrase. If the presenter can find a way to create such sound bites, the chances that the audience receive and act on your core message greatly increase. Here are some examples of sound bites:

- Design your design
- There is one way to succeed, and 90 ways to fail
- Take a bite-sized approach to dieting
- Vaccinations only work after being injected [1]

18.1.8 Briefly Reiterating Your Presentation

A very effective and frequently taken approach is the "three tells" method, namely

- Tell the audience what you are going to tell
- Tell it

- Tell them what they have been told

Research indicates that the maximum recall from hearing information is no more than 30%. The main reason the three tells is effective is because repetition gives multiple opportunities for an audience to grasp the message.

- Do not use dull phrases in your ending. Avoid, "so, to conclude" or "let me sum up".
- Appeal instead to the audience's need for relevance and meaning by asking rhetorical questions, such as "what effect does this have on how we act?" or "what result can you expect from doing this?" [1].

18.1.9 Use a Powerful Visual Image to End

- It is said that a picture is worth a thousand words. This saying is particularly correct with regard to presentations.
- Select an image which reflects the content of your presentation, whilst evoking the emotion which you wish the audience to feel afterwards. It may be a funny, inspiring or revealing image, as long as it fits your message. To take an example, a presentation about the benefits of prescribing antidepressants to women with postnatal depression might show the sun slowly emerging from behind dark clouds [1].

18.2   Reasons for Carefully Planning the Ending of a Presentation

A delicious dessert is the perfect way to end a celebratory meal. Afterwards, the guests only remember the delicious chocolate soufflé and forget all about the boring soup. The ending of a film, if it leaves us with a cliffhanger or another powerful emotion, keeps us wanting more. Likewise, a well-planned music concert ends with a rousing number, not an obscure study by a little-known composer. Adverts save the slogan for the end.

Given the fact that presentations also rely on the ending to leave an impression on the audience, it is surprising how often presentation endings fall flat. A slide with an irrelevant cartoon or a slide saying "thank you" are a disappointing way to end a presentation.

So, why is this the case? One explanation is that many presenters dislike or even hate presenting, since their fear of public speaking is so great. These types of presenters may be just desperate for the torture to end, so they can feel relieved at last. Since many audiences are also less than enthusiastic about what they are to hear, it may seem natural that presenters seek not to prolong an already painful experience.

However, this way of thinking is not fully rational. If you are to present successfully, you need to be inspirational and persuasive, and your presentation needs to finish in a similar way. After all, the maximum audience focus is usually at the beginning and end of a presentation. Thus the ending is the very best time to drive your central message home. Hitting the right emotional note at the end means the difference between success and failure.

18.3 Expert Techniques for Ending a Presentation

18.3.1 Be Brave Enough to Try Something Different

Think about any presentations you have attended in the past. Most likely you may struggle to recall the details of any of the presentation endings. Typically, there is a final slide with "thank you" written on it, but little else. This shows how hard it is to leave a final, decisive impression on an audience. The solution to this dilemma is to be as creative as possible and to be willing to try something new [2].

18.3.2 Do Not Leave the Ending to Chance

A common attitude amongst many inexperienced presenters is that the ending will flow naturally from the earlier part of their presentation. However, it is a mistake to leave such an important opportunity to be memorable to chance. No audience ever remembers a dull "Thank you. That's all". It risks undermining all the effort expended on the rest of the presentation. Time spent planning an ending is time well spent. It does not matter how many presentations you have done before, a planned ending will always outshine the most brilliant extempore performance. Treat the ending with the same respect as the rest of the presentation and plan exactly how to finish [2].

18.3.3 Prepare Your Presentation Backwards

It may seem paradoxical to begin preparing a presentation by concentrating on the ending first. However, this is one way to ensure that the crucial final stage has enough energy. If you start preparing from the beginning and work your way through to the end, there is a real danger that you will be tired by the time you come to the ending.

Presenters should always have their presenting objectives clearly in mind when preparing. Consider what the central message you wish to give really is. The structure of the presentation should then follow naturally on from these considerations [2].

18.3.4 Treat Your Presentation Like a Printed Book

Many presenters assume that the introduction to the presentation and the conclusion should be distinctly different. However, consider how a book is usually organised. The front and back cover often feature similar graphics and the blurb on the back cover generally talks about what the book contains. In the same way, the ending of a presentation can recapitulate some of the visual and text content of the introduction. You may want to pose a question at the beginning that you finally answer in the conclusion. Structuring a presentation in this way clearly defines the limits of the presentation and gives a satisfying sense of returning back to the beginning once more [2].

18.3.5 Avoid Telling the Audience It Will Soon Be Over

It is fairly common to hear presenters half-jokingly remark that the presentation is nearly over, "the torture is about to stop" or "you won't need to listen to me much longer". These kinds of remarks tend to be counterproductive. Rather than lightening the mood, they suggest to an audience that the presenter is fed up of presenting and that they can start thinking about something else instead. Why risk undermining your effort in this way?

Instead, presenters can signal the ending without the need to drop in tempo. If you use an expression like "this final point is especially worth considering" you signal to the audience that the climax of your presentation is coming and that they should pay even more attention than before. Of course, another solution is not to signal the end in advance at all. When the audience sees your summary and you explain what you want them to take away from the presentation, they can readily appreciate you are drawing to a close [2].

18.3.6 Keep the Finest Content Until the End

Use a storytelling approach to the presentation. Just as no novel or film gives away its ending straightaway, but rather builds suspense in the audience step-by-step, so you should save the most exciting part of the presentation until the end. Put the most convincing argument at the end. Or give a glimpse into a future full of promise as you conclude. Since the ending is the most easily remembered part of the presentation, your audience should remember the strongest statement of your message and the excitement of the ending [2].

18.3.7 Is It Worth Offering a Summary at the End?

Although many presentations do involve reiterating the main points at the end, this need not always be necessary. If the presentation takes the form of storytelling, a summary is usually not needed.

Nonetheless, in some cases it is helpful for the presenter to reiterate the main points and help set everything into context. Use the summary to remind your audience what you want them to remember and let them see how the details add up to the whole [2].

18.3.8 Make It Stick in People's Minds

Presentations have one characteristic in common with advertisements—the more they are memorable, the better they succeed. In a presentation, being memorable boils down to repetition. Repeated messages stick in the mind more easily and are remembered for longer. The ending is an opportunity to repeat the key content and fix it in your audience's memory. Some presenters like to make suggestions that will make the audience recall important details later, by saying something like: "As you travel home later, when you reach the traffic lights, try saying the warning system out loud".

You might also want to give some advice that may help your audience in other parts of their lives, too. For example, you may tell them that a memorisation technique you taught them to remember details of banking regulations is also valuable for remembering anniversaries and birthdays. If you connect with the audience as ordinary people, they will feel happier and relate better to the topic you have presented [2].

18.3.9 Pay Attention to Your Final Sentence

The final sentence you utter in a presentation is surprisingly important. It frequently happens that some audience members have lost their focus by the end of a presentation, but most people are actually back listening as you finish. Thus, make sure that the final sentence is something you want the audience to remember. Do not just trail off. It needs to be reflective of your central message and fit the emotion you want the audience to feel at the end [2].

The following are some recommendations on how to create an effective concluding sentence or sentences [2]:

- Your final message must be harmonious with the earlier content.
- Aim for brevity.
- Engage your audience's feelings. Let them feel positive, ready to take action and send them away thinking about what you have said. Consider using humour to make your point.
- You can reiterate a message or sound bite from earlier in the presentation and emphasise it at the end.
- There are various rhetorical techniques that make the message more memorable, such as the use of alliteration.
- If you present very often, you may wish to create a signature signing off phrase. This is quite common on YouTube channels, where many presenters have a particular catchphrase they end with, such as, "and that, folks, is history revisited".
- You can also end with a quote from a famous writer, if that helps to underline your message. Another option is to change a saying or proverb slightly, to provide an interesting and memorable twist. For example, in a presentation about health professionals taking part in sport, you might say, "An apple a day keeps the doctor in play".
- There are even other ways to end a presentation, such as displaying an evocative image or playing a brief, hard-hitting video clip.

18.3.10   Make the Audience Feel Part of Something Bigger

People enjoy the sense that they are involved in a greater shared purpose or activity. For this reason, it is good to end a presentation by emphasising harmonious intent and unified purpose. Substitute the first person plural (we, us) for the second person and first person singular (you, I) to highlight the shared purpose you have [2].

18.3.11   Maintain Your Professionalism All the Way Through

You must keep a professional air all the way through your presentation, which includes the ending. Do not feel you need to get the audience to approve or to apologise for any mistakes you may have made earlier. It is quite normal to occasionally trip up over your words or say something the wrong way round. The important thing is to accept you made a mistake, correct it if necessary, then carry on. You do not need to remind the audience of your mistakes in the conclusion. Audiences usually quickly forget about mistakes unless the presenter emphasises them.

Although it might seem obvious that emphasising your own shortcomings will not enhance your appearance of professionalism, many people have been brought up to act modestly and to admit freely when they are at fault. Being professional is not about denying you make mistakes but is about putting those errors in an appropriate perspective. Recognise the difference between true humility and professionalism and avoid too much self-criticism in public [2].

18.3.12 The End of the Presentation Means the Topic Is Finished

In many cases, the end of one topic means the beginning of another, fresh topic. However, do not take this approach when ending a presentation. Never introduce brand new material in the conclusion, as it will make your audience lose sight of the presentation's central message. In a situation where you realise you have left out an important point, it is better to omit it for now and perhaps send a correction by e-mail later.

This may not apply if there are questions and comments at the end of the slides. This type of interactive session is often suitable for mentioning new points [2].

18.3.13 Encourage Your Audience to Act After the Presentation

The ending is a good time to call on the audience to take action, whether that is to enrol for another presentation or to sign up for a product or service. If the timing is right, you can plug another service you offer in such a way that it seems only natural and very helpful to mention it at that point [2].

18.3.14 Move Seamlessly into the Comments and Questions

You should inform the audience at the outset of the presentation when they will have the opportunity to comment or ask questions. Where this is planned to occur straight after the presentation, ensure that you move seamlessly into the Q&As. Rather than asking if the audience has any questions, it is better for the presenter to throw out a question to the audience first and get the interaction started. By doing this, presenters can also maintain some control over the direction the Q&As take and ensure that the central message does not get overlooked [2].

18.3.15 The Last Slide

There are various opinions on what the ideal last slide should be like. Some presenters go for a simple one-word "end" or "questions?". Others feel that it is important to thank the audience for their time and attention, often in the form of a "thank you" slide. Whilst these are all reasonable options, using the last slide in this way represents a missed opportunity. You want the audience to leave in a pleasant mood and feeling specific emotions. The best final slide may not be text at all—why not show a cartoon, meme or striking image instead? Alternatively, some presenters may decide there is no need for a final slide, or perhaps it should be left blank. In this way, the momentum of the presentation can continue into the Q&As. You might signal the transition by saying something like: "So, now you have heard my perspective. I think it's time we heard your views" [2].

18.3.16   Should You Thank Your Audience?

There are also various viewpoints on whether presenters should say "thank you" to an audience or not. Some presentation experts believe expressing thanks is simply good etiquette. Other experts, however, see an expression of thanks as a cliché, which adds nothing to a presentation. Thus, the final decision on how to act lies with individual presenters. Of course, it is possible to thank your audience without putting the words on a slide. You can finish the presentation, then when the message has been clearly delivered, simply turn to the audience with a warm smile and thank them for their time.

18.3.17   Make It Personally Relevant

When you speak as an individual, the audience can relate to you and you can show genuine gratitude towards them. Say goodbye is a warm and friendly manner. The audience will remember you for longer. You might want to wish them a safe journey home. You can also add a personal note to the message of your presentation if you say something like: "I am looking forward to hearing what happens when you try out these new techniques in your own workplaces. Please let me know". Remember that presenters who are considered likeable are more effective at delivering messages than those who appear cold and aloof [2].

18.3.18   Avoid Rushing

Once the stress of speaking in public is over, it is natural for presenters to feel greatly relieved. Some presenters rush to clear away once the presentation is finished, gathering up their laptop and projector as quickly as possible to go home. This is another mistake, however, since the audience may perceive these actions as your wish to get away from them as soon as possible. Try instead to enjoy the recognition that comes from presenting and receive the audience approval with the warmth it deserves. You can always tidy up your equipment a little later. Do not rush to depart. You have worked hard for this moment.

A similar wish to get rid of the stress of public speaking may also underlie the tendency some presenters have to keep getting faster and faster. Be alert to how fast you are speaking and remember not to rush. Your audience will thank you for it.

18.3.19   Ensure Good Timekeeping

Nearly everyone who has ever attended a university lecture will be familiar with the experience of the audience noisily preparing to leave even before the lecture has concluded. This behaviour, whilst undoubtedly impolite, may be understandable when you consider that the students are balancing multiple other claims on their time, whether that is attending other lectures, practical classes or going to a part-time job. For everyone, time is a precious commodity. This is especially the case if you are presenting to an audience of busy professionals whose diaries may have very few gaps in them.

You can make life easier for your audience by sticking carefully to time. Calculate exactly how long each section of your presentation should take and make sure you do not over-run. You can practise timing by practising delivery, maybe in front of friends, relatives or sympathetic colleagues. You need to ensure that the time plan allows sufficient space to deliver each section at a comfortable pace, plus a little extra in case something goes wrong.

If you stick to time in this way, your audience will be able to give you their full attention, rather than worrying about being late for their next appointment. Not only will they feel less stressed, they will also retain your message better.

References

1. How to end a presentation to make a lasting impression (9 techniques). https://slideuplift.com/blog/business-powerpoint-presentations/how-to-end-a-presentation-to-make-a-lasting-impression-9-techniques/. Accessed 4 Oct 2021.
2. Because first impressions aren't everything: 20 tips and ideas to end your presentation in style. https://blog.presentationload.com/20-tips-end-presentation-in-style/. Accessed 4 Oct 2021.

19.1 Presenting as a Group

For presenters considering delivering a group presentation, there are several factors to consider to ensure success. The following are some points to bear in mind.

19.1.1 Select a Lead Presenter

The role of the lead presenter is to begin and conclude the presentation. It is therefore a key role. Usually the lead presenter is the most experienced member of the group or perhaps the presenter with the most confidence in public speaking. Some of the responsibilities this role entails are:

- Ensuring that the presentation attracts the full attention of the audience and gets them engaged from the very beginning.
- Performing introductions for each of the other presenters and explaining what part they play overall in the presentation.
- Guaranteeing a smooth transfer from presenter to presenter during delivery.
- Handling audience questions for any of the presenters, and signposting enquiries to the presenter most suited to address the issue.
- Providing a summary of the whole presentation and stating what action the presentation should lead to [1].

19.1.2 Ensure Cohesion Between the Various Sections

To guarantee that delivery by a group of presenters occurs in a smooth and cohesive fashion, decisions need to be made about the length of time to allocate to each presenter, how the segments should fit together and which presenter is responsible for

C. C. Cingi et al., *Improving Online Presentations*,
https://doi.org/10.1007/978-3-031-28328-4_19

each. These decisions may be taken by the group or by the lead presenter. Remember that time also needs to be allocated for Q&As.

There are several ways to map out a presentation. One is to use the Presentation Mapper methods marketed by Second Nature. A different approach is to lay out the presentation as a series of storyboards, using paper and pencil.

Avoid too detailed a view at the early planning stage. The key point to bear in mind is what the overall, central objectives of the presentation are, what part of the story each presenter will deliver and what the messages for the audience are. This then allows you to decide on the content. After the whole presentation has been storyboarded, decisions can then be taken on the length of each segment and the sections can start to be allocated to the different presenters.

As long as the initial planning stage is performed thoroughly, no time will be lost through unintended repetition by different presenters. It also guarantees there will be no gaps or inconsistencies which appear in the narration [1].

19.1.3 Make One Presenter Responsible for Slides Overall

For presentations where there are slides shown, one individual should be nominated to ensure the slide set has a consistent look and feel throughout. Graphics and text, as well as formatting, should be consistent and one person can put together slides produced by different presenters to ensure this is the case. A consistent slide set creates a positive impression of professionalism and attention to detail [1].

19.1.4 Set Aside Time for Practice

Ensuring that the presentation delivery is well-rehearsed is essential for success. This allows you to decide on where the presenters can sit whilst waiting to present, and their movements when they come to deliver their section. You will need to consider where your audience will be and how best to utilise the venue you have selected. A solution that works very well is to arrange your presenters from left-to-right in order of delivery, with the lead presenter in the middle. This then confirms the audience's usual expectations of reading from left to right, which means that the order will appear intuitive.

There are several techniques which make the best use of movement during presentations and which show how to control the space as you present.

By practising well, each presenter has the opportunity to craft a confident and polished delivery.

As long as the presentation has a clear and interesting central thread that ties everything together, the presenters can smoothly pass the baton on, and everyone keeps to time, the presentation should be a success. Rehearsal ensures this becomes a reality. A rehearsal also lets presenters practise responding to different questions and comments which may come up in the Q&As.

It is especially valuable to have a neutral third party observe the rehearsal, to provide the audience viewpoint and guarantee that the presentation appears logical and coherent and the time plan is closely adhered to. In an ideal world, this third party would be someone with expertise in coaching presenters since he or she can then give each presenter advice and feedback on delivery. A more usual situation is one in which a senior colleague offers to fulfil this role, offering constructive criticism and giving the benefit of his or her own experience [1].

19.1.5 Getting Ready on the Day of Actual Delivery

Having insufficient time to prepare to present as a group is a disaster waiting to happen. It is essential to ensure the technical equipment is working correctly and usable before the presentation is due to begin. Where a group is presenting in an unfamiliar environment, or a venue to which they do not normally have access, it is best to ensure access is available at least half an hour before the presentation, so that everything can be got ready on time.

Furthermore, where the venue is unfamiliar, the presenters can utilise any time before the presentation accustoming themselves to the layout, such as any restrictions on movement, where tripping hazards may occur, what the audience can see from various angles and how the acoustics work. It is useful to work out what sort of distractions may occur, such as noise from a nearby meeting room or the sound of cars passing [1].

19.1.6 Presenters Should Support Each Other

It is very disheartening for a presenter participating in a group presentation to see the other team members appear bored. No matter how often you have seen and heard your colleagues' presentations during rehearsals, show that you still feel excited and interested by what they have to say. Encourage them by smiling, nodding or laughing at the gags. When the audience sees the other presenters acting in this way, they take their cue from them and act with the same level of engagement.

19.1.7 Achieving Maximum Benefit from the Experience

Presentations delivered as a group are not very frequently undertaken, but when they do occur, they represent an excellent opportunity for group learning. One way to ensure that the experience yields maximum value is for the group to meet the next day after the presentation and carry out a "post-presentation review", focusing on where the presentation succeeded and any potential areas for improvement. This review should encompass the follow questions:

- How successfully were things done prior to the presentation itself?
- How was the equipment used?
- Was the message clear and did the presentation flow smoothly?
- How much detail was included?
- How well was time kept to, both overall and within each presenter's segment?
- How well did the transitions between presenters go?
- How were Q&As dealt with?
- Did the team support each other non-verbally during delivery?
- How did each presenter deliver? Did everyone speak confidently?

19.2   Presenting More Effectively as a Group

Many presenters feel unsure how to begin when they are asked to take part in a group presentation. Group presentations are often prone to failure because no particular individual takes on overall responsibility for the group presentation. It is common to assume that, if the individual presenters produce a good presentation, the overall presentation will automatically be of high quality. This, however, is a far from correct assumption.

Group presentations have the unique characteristic that they involve more than one presenter, but, just like all other types of presentation, to be successful they need to demonstrate cohesion, have a structure that includes an introductory and concluding segment, and exhibit thematic unity [2].

Steps leading to more effective group presentations [2]:

- **Engage Your Audience from the Outset:** Effective presentations attract the interest of the audience right from the start. Group presentations must also achieve this, by having a powerful introduction.
- **Provide Introductions for All the Presenters:** Ensure that the introduction explains who each of the presenters is.
- **Include Transition Sections:** When presenters finish their sections they should explain they are handing over to the next presenter, so that the transition is smooth. They may say something like: "Now, Peter will explain to us how Currency Swaps work in practice. Over to you, Peter". This should then be acknowledged by the next speaker: "Thanks, Jessica".
- **Include Movement:** The presenter currently in the "hot seat" should move to the middle of the stage or towards the front, providing visual clarity about exactly who is speaking at the time.
- **Use Visuals Correctly:** Make sure that presenters are looking at the audience, not the visuals, as they present.
- **Other Presenters Can Assist with the Slides:** In group presentations, the current presenter should not be hidden behind a laptop or lectern. If required, other presenters can operate the laptop on behalf of the speaker.
- **Incorporate Pauses at Strategic Intervals:** In individual presentations, being too hasty when presenting creates many problems. The tendency to rush is ampli-

fied in group presentations. To counteract this tendency, incorporate pauses and make a deliberate effort to allow some silence. There is no need for every second to be filled with a presenter's voice.

- **Presenters Should Listen to Each Other Attentively:** If the presenters look as if they find the presentation dull, the audience will certainly consider it boring. Presenters who are not currently speaker should appear to be engaged and actively listening, supplying non-verbal feedback to the speaker. This then encourages similar behaviour and engagement from the audience members.
- **Provide a Clear Conclusion:** There should be a concluding section where the key facts and concepts are reiterated and conclusions expressed. The ending is vital to providing cohesion and thematic integrity in a group presentation.
- **Practise, Practise, Practise:** Run through the entire presentation a minimum of three times. The presenters need to work together as a team and should be familiar with any cues from each other that they need to speak. The presentation should be practised until delivery is fluent and without awkward gaps.

19.3   Factors that Make Group Presentations Highly Successful

19.3.1 Four Key Actions to Take

The following four key actions are needed:

1. Analyse the topic carefully and be completely familiar with it
   (a) Ask yourself, "What is the objective in presenting this topic?"
   (b) Ensure you know exactly what the topic should be.
   (c) Be clear about what relevance the topic has for your intended audience.
2. Analyse your audience. Know who they are.
   (a) Think about the demographic characteristics of the audience (age, gender balance, cultural factors, etc.)
   (b) Select examples that really speak to that demographic.
   (c) Use language that fits the topic, but avoid lapsing into technicalese.
   (d) If you use a particular word, ensure you pronounce it in a way your audience can recognise.
3. Analyse the presenting group. Understand the strong and weak points, both individually and as a group.
   (a) Presenters with confidence in public speaking are suitable for the introductory and concluding sections.
   (b) Technical experts are better for discussion sections.
   (c) Q&As are best handled by presenters who think well on their feet.
4. Practice makes perfect.
   One of the main aims in practising is to produce a cohesive, united presentation.

19.3.2 Craft a UNIFIED Presentation

- The group need to collaborate to ensure there is a single, unifying structure to the presentation, i.e. a single introductory section, body and concluding remarks.
- One presenter has the responsibility for assembling the slides into a single deck.
- The slides need a consistent look and feel all the way through.
- Individual presenters may create their own slides, but these are then adapted to the group style by the slide co-ordinator.
- In group work of this kind, everyone is responsible for technical accuracy, avoiding typos, etc.
- Use language that reflects group work. It is better to use the first person plural rather than the singular (i.e. "we" not "I").
- Collaborate so that the central argument and message is as compelling as possible.
- Ensure that slides, and segments presented by different speakers, follow smoothly on from each other. Do this by consciously linking each subtopic to the previous ones presented. Each time a new presenter speaks, that person should be introduced and their topic area outlined. It is more straightforward if presenters treat the topics as having a degree of overlap, rather than as completely distinct matters [3].

19.3.3 Every Presenter Should Dress Appropriately

Group presenters should dress similarly, although there is no requirement for them to choose identical outfits. The dress style (generally fairly formal) should reflect the professional image the group wishes to project [3].

19.3.4 Advice on Delivering the Presentation

- The opening section of the presentation should include an introduction of the group presenters.
- One slide should offer a preview of the topics to be discussed.
- During rehearsal, check every slide for any spelling mistakes, inconsistencies or errors.
- The practice run-through should be exactly like it will be with an audience present.
- Get the presenters to constructively criticise each other.
- Avoid standing holding speech cue cards. If you use them, place them where you can refer to them.
- Turn your back to the screen and always face the audience whilst you are speaking.

- Ensure that your body language signals the same thing you are saying verbally. Inconsistent body language is very confusing for audiences. For example, do not describe an unpleasant or painful situation whilst grinning from ear to ear.
- Gesturing with the hands is helpful but should not be at a distracting level [3].

References

1. Huckle B. What are some effective group presentation methods or skills. 2021. https://www.secondnature.com.au/blog/effective-group-presentation-methods-or-skills/. Accessed 4 Oct 2021.
2. 10 tips for improving group presentations. 2021. https://jamcarthur.com/2011/11/01/10-tips-for-improving-group-presentations/. Accessed 4 Oct 2021.
3. Elements of effective group presentations. https://www.siue.edu/artsandsciences/acs/SpeechCenter/EffectiveGroup.shtml. Accessed 4 Oct 2021.

The Deadly Sins and Cardinal Virtues of Online Presentations

20.1 What to Do and Not to Do When Presenting Virtually

20.1.1 *Do* Utilise Visuals More Extensively

Slides which consist of text alone, or where the same visual appears over and over again, tend to bore audiences. Remember to maintain visual variety and interest.

20.1.2 *Do* Use Graphics to Highlight the Main Idea on a Slide

Don't forget to let graphical elements guide your audience in seeing the key information on a slide. Ensure they cannot miss the point.

20.1.3 *Do* Make Time for the Audience to Ask Questions

When presenting virtually, do allow for some level of interactivity with your audience. Have section breaks where the audience can ask their questions. This is much better than saving all the questions until the end, by which time your audience may have lost interest.

20.1.4 *Do* Have a Backup Plan, Just in Case

If anything can go wrong, it will go wrong, as they say. This affects online presentations, too. Remember to keep backup copies of your slide set on a separate flash disk, portable hard disk and in the cloud. A file can easily become corrupted and unusable or get accidentally deleted.

© The Author(s), under exclusive license to Springer Nature Switzerland AG 2023
C. C. Cingi et al., *Improving Online Presentations*,
https://doi.org/10.1007/978-3-031-28328-4_20

20.1.5 *Don't* Forget to Print a Copy for Reference

You can print out the slides onto paper to make it easier to find the slide you want in response to questions or comments. The slides are much easier to see in this format and, once you know the slide number, you can jump straight to that slide.

20.1.6 *Do* Ensure You Rehearse Well

Online presentations rely on two technologies working in tandem—the slide application (such as PowerPoint) and the teleconferencing application (such as Zoom). Rehearse using both technologies together, so that you can handle any situations you are likely to encounter [1].

20.2 Fatal Flaws in Virtual Presentations

20.2.1 Being Too Slow to Address the Main Issue

Currently, audience attention spans are getting ever shorter and time is a luxury few of us now possess. Therefore, make your point succinctly and without unnecessary delay. Whether you are making a sales pitch, launching a product or seeking consensus on an issue, aim for brevity and a punchy message. Outline the message in few words and make the meaning as crystal clear as possible. Let the structure of your presentation allow for maximum clarity and use evidence to support, justify and strengthen your argument [2].

20.2.2 Too Much Text

When a presentation is delivered face-to-face, the attention of the audience is divided between the presenter and the slides. If the slides contain a large volume of text, the audience are free to focus on the presenter's words and body language instead. However, in online presentations, the main thing the audience sees is the slide. All the visual focus is on one thing. Therefore, text-dense slides really stand out. Don't make your audience wade through mountains of text and dense thickets of bullet points to see the message! Keep slides concise and easy to remember. Avoid typos and ensure consistency in font size, font type and colour scheme. To communicate effectively, a brief, highly relevant and clear message is absolutely essential.

20.2.3 Cramming the Information onto Too Few Slides

We are so used to being advised to cut down the number of slides in a presentation that it may be a shock to hear that some presenters actually use too few slides. The main problem in such cases is that of putting too much information on each slide. The slides then become very crowded and difficult to understand. It is far better to spread the information out, so that the relationship between the different points is clearer. When there is less on each slide, the audience feel the presentation is moving quickly enough to keep their interest. Slides that indicate the overall structure, such as division into sections, are also very valuable in helping the audience to follow the overall direction [2].

20.2.4 Insufficient Visuals

Visual imagery is the single element most capable of enhancing the impact of a presentation and increasing the audience engagement. Not only do visuals provide an attractive appearance to a slide, they also assist with comprehension of the message. After all, it is estimated that 65% of individuals are primarily visual learners. The images you use should be high quality and visually appealing. Shutterstock has an excellent collection of images that illustrate concepts or symbolise ideas, whereas Unsplash goes for more realistic and royalty-free images. Do not hide an image in the corner of a slide—let it fill the whole slide and tell its message clearly [2].

20.2.5 Not Making Full Use of Your Voice

The biggest mistake of all is to just read off the slides as though you were a text-to-sound converter! Reading aloud is around 40% slower than reading silently. In educated adults, the average silent reading speed is 280 words each minute, whereas on average the reading aloud rate is 173 words per minute. This difference is especially apparent in an online presentation, making some presenters seem to be moving at a snail's pace. Rather than reading off the slide, it is much more effective to talk around the slide, supplying extra meaning with examples or other facts. The tone of voice also plays a major role in how the audience perceive the presentation. A lively, enthusiastic tone generates that emotion in the audience. You need to use your diaphragm to give power to your voice, so either stand up or sit upright. Vary the speed and tone, pausing from time to time. Remember that the audience are deprived of many of the usual body language clues that enhance meaning, so, just like a radio presenter, you need to make full use of your voice to bring out the full meaning [2].

20.2.6 Doing Everything Yourself

Another very serious error to avoid in a virtual presentation is talking all the time, without letting the audience say anything. In face-to-face meetings, it is harder for people to get distracted by messages on their telephone or by social media updates than it is online, where no one can see if an audience member decides to ignore the presentation and look at the headlines instead. One way to combat this tendency for audience members to zone out is to incorporate regular interaction with the audience. These interactions should be timed to occur at 5- or 6-min intervals and can be in the form of polls, surveys, questions or requests for feedback. Interaction may occur via chat or by handing over the microphone. There are several applications that help to set up quizzes or polls, such as Mentimeter, Kahoot or Quizizz. If you decide to open the chat box, it can rapidly become distracting. Therefore, it is best to appoint a chat moderator who can respond. If a presentation is very long, dividing it up amongst two presenters may help to provide some much-needed variety. The more variety there is, the more likely you are to retain your audience's attention [2].

20.2.7 You Fail to Put Together a Contingency Plan

There is a great deal of truth in the idea that if something can go wrong, it eventually will do so. There are many technical issues that can occur, including non-working microphones or video cameras, inability to share screen or sound, applications closing unexpectedly, unresponsive computers and unscheduled system restarts. Then there are the totally unanticipated things that can happen during a presentation, like a couple having a major, noisy row in the next door office or water dripping through the ceiling. In all such circumstances, disaster can hopefully be averted if you have a contingency plan. The plan should include backup copies of your presentation, including in an easy-to-share format, such as portable document format (pdf). Always remain calm if something does go wrong. The audience are probably less surprised than you might imagine. After all, technical failure has become very familiar to most people since the major shift to online presentations and remote working first took place [2].

20.2.8 Insufficiently Trained Presenter

Perhaps the majority of presenters have never undertaken formal training on how to present. However, even a fairly basic level of professional training can give a significant advantage to a presenter. Learning about tricks expert presenters use, trying out different methods and getting well-informed feedback on your performance all help to make a more effective presenter, able to persuade audiences and produce memorable and enjoyable presentations. Just as there is a difference between a keen amateur cook and a professional chef, so a certain level of training can elevate a presenter's performance from ordinary to extraordinary [2].

20.3   How to Avoid a Presentation Catastrophe

The following are some tips on how to avoid a presentation disaster.

20.3.1 First Fatal Error: Acting Like a Presentation Robot

Appropriate body language is a vital part of presenting, whether you present from a sitting or standing position. Indeed, body language is arguably even more important in virtual than face-to-face presentations, because there already exist barriers between the presenter and audience. Effective body language helps to overcome the distance, but this requires conscious effort in an online setting. Presenters need to act even more energetically than usual, and with more distinct gestures. To see the level of exaggeration required, try recording yourself delivering the presentation in two different ways—once with no special attention to body language, then by consciously attending to gestures, etc. You can then calibrate your body language, depending on which version appears more natural and spontaneous. Some presenters suggest keeping presenting quirks that they use in face-to-face events in the online event. If you normally chuckle as you recall an amusing event, keep doing so. If you would normally undo your tie and sip from your morning coffee, continue to do so, as your audience may find you more human and relatable. There are limits on gesture and movement in a virtual presentation due to the camera's limitations, but within the space the camera can capture, be sure to convey your abundant enthusiasm and energy, so that the audience do not want to take their eyes off you [3].

20.3.2 Second Fatal Error: Lack of Eye Contact

It is not easy to make convincing eye contact in an online presentation. In face-to-face presentations, skilful presenters generally make near-constant eye contact with different audience members in different parts of the room. This is obviously harder to achieve online. Many online presenters find it awkward to look at their own image on the screen in front of them, so tend to turn away from the camera. This is a mistake. It is usually possible to turn off display of your own image, but the main issue is that presenters need to look into the camera in order to appear to be making eye contact. So, rather than moving around the room, you should look directly into the camera from time to time to convey the impression of eye contact. One helpful tip for presenters who may forget to do this is to place a small smiley sticker next to the camera, to remind them to glance in that direction and smile [3].

20.3.3 Third Fatal Error: Too Lengthy a Presentation

One key consideration when presenting online is that audiences generally have a shorter attention span than in a face-to-face event. Accordingly, presentations need to be made briefer. Some experts consider a 10 min online presentation to require a similar concentration effort to 20 min face-to-face. Just as in a sporting event where players can only hold the ball for a limited period before passing it, so presenters should be limited in how long they can speak before interacting or changing topic, in order to maintain presenting momentum. Online content needs to be rendered more "bite-size" than usual to give the audience the best chance to absorb the message. In practice, producing bite-sized content means simplifying slides so that they contain just one or two principal points, making extensive use of visuals and only commenting where something is especially pertinent or interesting [3].

20.3.4 Fourth Fatal Error: Failure to Rehearse

Rehearsing your presentation prior to the actual delivery is not merely advisable, it is essential to avoid a presenting disaster. Presenting online involves controlling both the slide software (such as PowerPoint) and the videoconferencing application (such as Zoom or Microsoft Teams). Thus, presenters need to be thoroughly familiar with the way the software and computer works, as well as the dynamics of interaction with online audiences. Even if you do remember that a poll is needed before presenting a particular slide, it is vital that you also know how to carry out the poll in a way that does not cause an agonising delay in presentation delivery. The absolute best way to do a rehearsal is to use the same set up as on the day of actual delivery and to get several friends or colleagues to log on as a virtual audience for you to interact with. This kind of rehearsal is always beneficial [3].

References

1. Online presentation do's and don'ts. https://www.deccatalkingpoints.com/online-presentation-dos-and-donts/. Accessed 4 Oct 2021.
2. The 8 killer mistakes to avoid when presenting online. https://www.readmatthews.com/2020/10/20/the-8-common-mistakes-of-online-presenting/. Accessed 4 Oct 2021.
3. Brownlee D. Presenting virtually? Don't make these 5 tragic virtual presentation mistakes. https://www.forbes.com/sites/danabrownlee/2020/05/17/presenting-virtually-dont-make-these-5-tragic-virtual-presentation-mistakes/?sh=1d6000e9234d. Accessed 4 Oct 2021.

Dealing with Challenging Presenting Situations 21

21.1 Problems When Presenting

21.1.1 Giving Unwelcome News

A presenter may occasionally need to give unwelcome news to an audience involving a decision they will not agree with. The objective in such a situation is to be informative about the decision but not to show either personal agreement or disagreement at that stage. In communication theory, this approach is referred to as "fogging". The audience realise you are acknowledging the facts but not discussing the merits of the decision. They should also realise that discussion will occur at a later stage, once everyone is in full possession of the facts [1]. Fogging involves two stages.

21.1.1.1 Stage 1
You acknowledge that the audience may have powerful feelings about the information, but stress that you are merely providing information at this point.

21.1.1.2 Stage 2
Having set the ground rules for the presentation, you go on to supply the related facts [1].

21.1.2 Delivering Unwelcome News to Groups

Avoid the temptation to skirt around the issue and to supply some form of apology or justification. Make sure you stick to the facts and explain them clearly and succinctly.

You may say something like, "The purpose of this meeting is to inform you that ten individuals are being made redundant this week".

© The Author(s), under exclusive license to Springer Nature
Switzerland AG 2023
C. C. Cingi et al., *Improving Online Presentations*,
https://doi.org/10.1007/978-3-031-28328-4_21

Respond to an angry reaction by listening carefully and without speaking yourself. Do not attempt to express your own feelings. If members of the audience begin to cry, be patient waiting for them to gather themselves. Once you have supplied the necessary facts, avoid giving further details until the emotions have settled in the room. Allow the audience the opportunity to state how they feel before you supply them with the extra details you need them to know.

Express your understanding of the audience's response by saying something like, "I can clearly see how much of a shock this has been. Your anger is easy to understand".

The only way your audience will be receptive to receiving further information is if you have given them the opportunity to vent their emotions and have demonstrated some empathy with their emotions. Provided this has been achieved, you can carry on to the next stage, such as supplying information about a redundancy package.

At this point, you may be able to involve the audience in some part of the decision, such as what format the redundancy announcement will take. However, be careful that you do not offer to involve the audience in matters to which they cannot be allowed to contribute [1].

21.1.3 Dealing with Questions of a Hostile or Aggressive Nature

21.1.3.1   General Strategy
- Keep calm and remain rational.
- Demonstrate that you understand and have an interest in answering the question.
- Attempt to find some common ground contained in the remarks made by the questioner.

21.1.4 Different Tactics in Answering

Consider getting the questioner to supply some background to the question. This may expose weaknesses in the questioner's rationale, which you can then address.

If you ask the questioner to be more specific in what they say, you can address a particular situation without the risk of the situation escalating into a stand-off.

You may need to ask what the question is driving at to be able to supply an adequate answer. In seeking clarification, you may also expose some assumption or unjustified inference that the questioner has made which you can then exploit to justify your own position.

21.1.5 The Approach to Answering

Supply an answer that is rational and clearly states your view. Try to be specific rather than discussing generalities.

Ensure that you do not get drawn into a slanging match or a situation where subjective opinions are seen to clash.

Reply in an assertive manner, but do not stray into becoming aggressive yourself [1].

21.1.6 What Not to Do

Do not allow yourself to start arguing. Rather than confronting the questioner, take a more neutral approach (i.e. use the fogging technique discussed earlier). If you cannot establish common ground, then agree to respect each other's opinion.

Do not try to bluff your way out. It is better to acknowledge the limits of your knowledge.

Do not attack the questioner. Remain professional, respectful and polite. Avoid the urge to quash the question through a sarcastic response [1].

21.2 Twelve Methods to Use in Dealing with Problems When Presenting

The following sections discuss some of the causes for audience hostility or a lack of receptiveness and offer techniques to deal with these issues.

Potential Issues
- An audience may strongly reject the content of your presentation if there is a feeling that what you suggest will harm their interests.
- Audiences may not comprehend the message and therefore not accept it.
- People may feel bound to their previous way of thinking or acting and reject attempts to change the situation.
- Audiences may question whether you are sufficiently knowledgeable to challenge their own beliefs.
- People may feel disinterested and detached from the issues you are describing.
- There may be a limit on how far the audience can perceive the bigger picture. They may be blinkered in their views.
- They may exclusively focus on negative aspects, ignoring any potential advantages.

If an audience attending a presentation suffers from one of these issues, the presenter will be faced with an extremely difficult task. In extreme circumstances, the audience may be openly hostile. In any case, these issues make the audience less receptive and may mean they disengage altogether. Clearly, this is a situation that will interfere with effective delivery of a presentation unless successfully addressed.

Fortunately, however, there are a number of ways that presenters can deal with these kinds of problematic situation. Twelve techniques or attitudes to adopt for managing problematic audiences have been identified, as follows [2].

21.2.1 Be Able to View a Problem from Various Angles

If you face an audience who are likely to reject or disagree with your message and the content of your presentation, one key technique is to ensure you understand in detail how the issue must look from your audience's viewpoint. Being passionate about your presentation, believing what you say and speaking well are all important, but the key issue in such a situation is that the audience have a different viewpoint. You will need to empathise with their viewpoint and comprehend how they have reached their ideas.

In fact, the inability to see an issue from another perspective is one factor in why such a situation may arise. Be sure to think the topic through carefully from other perspectives before you deliver your material, and that will give you the confidence to anticipate and deal with challenges [2].

21.2.2 Identify the Weak Points and Patch Them

Getting ready to face a potentially unreceptive or hostile audience should include noting any weak points in the presentation and being prepared to justify your overall argument, despite these weaknesses. It is sounder to acknowledge any limitations than to deny they exist. However, acknowledgement of weaknesses should be accompanied by an explanation of how the weaknesses are to be addressed. Your audience may well still reject your message, but they will respect the fact that you are thinking about their concerns.

Alongside a thorough knowledge of potential weaknesses in your presentation, a knowledge of your own personal weak points is just as necessary. Think of what your own triggers are, then plan how you can stop these triggers causing you to lose control of the event [2].

21.2.3 Look Out for the Snipers

It pays to find out who the most challenging individuals are ahead of time. There are some people who seem to delight in "sniping", in other words, deliberately trying to put you off. They frequently sit towards the back and attack like a sniper from this hidden position. If possible, try to speak in a friendly way with such individuals before the presentation, so that you can reduce their initial hostility. They may even appreciate you reaching out to them and giving them some recognition.

Do not retaliate if the sniper attacks you. Remain undistracted and focused. Thank them for the question or feedback, add extra support to your argument and continue with the next slide.

Snipers generally want to make you get angry and distract you from your presentation [2]. If you remain calm and do not rise to their bait, the presentation will be more successful.

21.2.4 Do Not Take It Personally

In the majority of cases where an audience is hostile or otherwise unreceptive, it is rarely a question of the audience having personal animosity towards the presenter. Do not fall into the trap of thinking difficult questions or hostile comments are designed to attack you as an individual. Indeed, whoever presents to certain audiences, there is likely to be a cold reception. Separate your personal feelings from the issue and see it as a professional challenge, presenting as well as possible in a difficult environment. Unfortunately, many people forget the adage, "Do not shoot the messenger". However, as a professional, your duty is to deliver the message as clearly and persuasively as possible, whilst also accepting that the audience's viewpoint may be quite different from your own [2].

21.2.5 Establish Ground Rules First

You, as the presenter, are responsible for the presentation, so it is a good idea to establish your authority at the beginning.

The following are suggested ground rules:

The audience should turn phones to silent and not answer them during the presentation.
State when there will be the opportunity to feedback and ask questions.
Explain that you will be the person responsible for the timing, the topics to be discussed, handling feedback and all the presenting equipment [2].

21.2.6 Reduce Negative Emotions in the Room

- A smile diffuses a lot of tension. If there are suitable occasions to do so, inject a note of humour. Humour also diffuses tension
- Avoid replying to comments in a defensive or negative manner.
- Try to stay on ground where there is clear evidence to decide. Avoid excessive speculation.
- Try to see the issue from the audience's eyes and show empathy for their viewpoint [2].

21.2.7 Meet the Audience's Needs

Everybody always has a need of some kind and it is human nature to try to resolve our own unmet needs. Audiences who feel their needs are not being met may respond in an ill-tempered, unresponsive or hostile way. This may be the issue with a challenging audience, in which case you should do whatever you can to make sure that you meet the audience's needs as far as possible.

The kinds of unmet needs typically encountered include:

- More factual detail, evidence to back up a theory or example where it applies.
- The need to feel respected, acknowledged and understood.
- The need to participate, by interaction and involvement.
- The need to feel emotionally connected to the presenter and topic [2].

21.2.8 Make Friends Not Enemies

On occasion, presenters may deliver to an audience in which there is a person with a greater knowledge of the subject who feels the need to make his or her opinion heard. Such experts may come across as confrontational unless you simply acknowledge they are worth listening to and allow them to make some kind of comment.

At the same time, ensure that other members of the audience also have the chance to comment, so that no one is left feeling excluded. It is better to make allies out of people who wish to speak than turning them into your enemies by forcing them to remain silent [2].

21.2.9 What to Do if the Audience Begin to Yawn

It is sometimes the case that audiences are not as attentive as a presenter might wish. Some individuals may check their smartphones during the presentation, glance repeatedly at their watches or begin yawning. You may even observe people whispering to each other. In such a situation, it is important not to succumb to a feeling of panic, fuelled by the suspicion you have lost your audience. It is important to realise that many people perform such actions all the time, without necessarily doing so out of boredom or a lack of interest. Thus, feeling you have lost an audience due to such signs is an unjustified conclusion and there is no need to panic in such a situation [2].

21.2.10 Demonstrate Humility

Whenever you present, aim to be authoritative, but not authoritarian. The former indicates that you are professional and knowledgeable. The latter indicates arrogance and will make you enemies [2].

21.2.11 Hold a Council of War First

If you anticipate difficulties, it is highly advisable to hold a meeting before the day of the presentation with colleagues who can help you iron out any potential problems by undertaking the following tasks:

Firstly, gather everyone's opinions on what questions or objections might potentially be voiced during the presentation and plan the best way to answer.
Secondly, perform role plays to allow the presenter to feel they have the skills necessary to deal with any of the anticipated challenges [2].

21.2.12 The Way You Respond to Questions Is Key

Answering questions and responding to comments is frequently a source of anxiety to presenters. Indeed, it is the number one most feared part of the whole presenting activity. Many presenters have the sense that their ignorance may be revealed by questions from the audience, and that this will result in the audience having a poor opinion about the presenter. Such fears are, however, exaggerated. It is practically impossible for one particular individual to have all the answers to every potential question at their fingertips. Nor do audiences expert such an unrealistic level of expertise from a presenter. However, in order to deal successfully with questions in a way that enhances rather than detracts from your reputation, there are certain approaches which should be followed.

In the first place, avoid the temptation to bluster your way out of a situation in which you genuinely do not know the answer. Such bluffing is very obvious and creates an unfavourable impression. Conversely, there is no need to be excessively apologetic about not knowing the answer, either. The best approach is to thank the questioner, say that you currently lack the necessary information to answer the question fully and offer to get back with the answer once you have done the necessary research. It goes without saying that such a promise must be fulfilled if you wish to maintain a reputation for professionalism.

Whilst answering questions, look at everybody in the room, not simply the questioner. By making eye contact with multiple people, you involve them in the answer, whereas if you only make eye contact with the questioner, other members of the audience may feel detached from the whole process, or even ignored.

It is often a good idea to ask the audience for their own opinion, if you face particularly hard questions.

When someone is asking a question, ensure that you listen carefully to everything the person is saying and do not rush to provide your response. In many cases, a presenter feels anxious about questions and rushes to give an answer, without fully comprehending what the questioner wants to know. Conquer the urge to speak and be patient as the question is being asked. If the question is unclear, be prepared to get the questioner to explain exactly what they want to know.

Avoid introducing a negative air into your responses. It is unwise to antagonise the questioner by rubbishing his or her suggestion or dismissing the comment as incorrect.

Likewise, do not take the approach that the majority of presenters take in flattering the questioner by saying something like: "Wow! Great question!" This rarely sounds genuine and may even suggest you are humouring the questioner. Another problem with doing this is that it compels you to say the same to everyone, unless you want them to feel their questions were somehow less valid or less worth asking.

In dealing with any of the challenging situations described in this chapter, receiving some training and practising your response will build your confidence and the ability to overcome the problem. Unless you only present very rarely, it is highly likely that eventually you will find yourself in a similar problematic situation. The 12 strategies outlined here can be refined and developed to cope in every situation. The main point to remember is always to stay calm and to keep control of your emotions. In this way you will remain in charge and able to deliver high quality presentations, whatever the circumstances [2].

References

1. Handling challenging presentation situations. 2021. https://www.trainingcoursematerial. com/free-training-articles/presentation-skills/handling-challenging-presentation-situations. Accessed 4 Oct 2021.
2. Decastro M. 12 Tactics for handling challenging public speaking situations. 2015. https://mindfulpresenter.com/challenging-public-speaking/. Accessed 4 Oct 2021.

Communication in Healthcare

22.1 Introduction

The way that doctors and other healthcare practitioners interact and communicate with patients has a highly significant effect upon how patients evaluate the care they have been given [1, 2]. There is an abundance of evidence demonstrating that clinicians who communicate effectively achieve better outcomes both for the patients and the teams within which they work. Patients relate well to certain healthcare professionals, and this then translates into better involvement in treatment decision-making, higher levels of concordance and more effective management of their own condition by patients [3–9].

22.2 Communicative Modalities Employed in Healthcare

When the literature relating to healthcare communication is reviewed, it is evident that written forms of communication predominate, despite the fact that face-to-face communication is generally considered ideal. The literature also demonstrates that there is general agreement on what benefits written communication in healthcare is able to offer [9].

The richest type of communication, however, involves face-to-face contact. Only in such situations can each party observe the body language and facial expressions employed, which adds an extra dimension of meaning to the words used. Prior to the advent of modern communicative technologies, face-to-face communication could only occur in the physical presence of the other party. Now, however, certain technologies are able to replicate aspects of face-to-face communication, even though the parties are physically distant from each other [10]. Videoconferencing is one such example. Despite the availability of such technologies, it appears that face-to-face communication is in decline, with healthcare professionals increasingly preferring indirect methods of communication to direct ones [11]. E-mail, which can be

C. C. Cingi et al., *Improving Online Presentations*,
https://doi.org/10.1007/978-3-031-28328-4_22

set up to provide a "read" receipt, is seen as an effective alternative to speaking on the telephone or in person whilst also allowing an audit trail to be established [1, 9].

Indeed, written communication, understood to include e-mail, letters, fax, etc. is the dominant, and often the sole, way that many healthcare practitioners communicate between themselves [12]. The format of the majority of written messages falls into two categories: referral letters and discharge documentation. The former consists of three subtypes, namely requests for particular forms of assessment or investigation, or treatment, requests for a second opinion and requests to share the management of a case [13]. Discharge documentation typically concerns the situation where a patient is being discharged from a healthcare facility. However, discharge documentation may also relate to other situations, e.g. a specialist answering a general physician's questions about a patient who was never actually admitted to hospital. The complexity of discharge documentation may create issues with what particular terms refer to, since many of the expressions used hark back to an era when care was mostly provided to admitted patients rather than the current situation where outpatient clinics see the most patients [9].

There are undoubted benefits from communicating in written form, such as the fact that it enables the documentation to be reviewed at a later date and the ease with which written communications can be shared amongst the professionals involved in a patient's care [14]. Written documentation not only serves a communicative but also a medicolegal purpose [15]. Additionally, the digital environment in which healthcare now occurs permits written communication to be near-instantly available, which enhances its value yet further [16].

Letters may also serve an educational purpose, by supplying more detailed information of value in appreciating the complexities of a case, such as prognosis, likely complications and the alternative ways in which it can be managed [17]. This educational aspect is more apparent in letters drafted by specialists than those written by general practitioners [18]. Some 25% of letters by specialists were deemed educational by one study, compared to 3% of those by general practitioners [17].

22.3 Inefficient Written Communication

The literature contains many studies on how written communication may become inefficient. Research which took a cross-sectional approach and sampled from various countries and healthcare environments demonstrates a high degree of consensus about what constitutes ideally effective written communication and how written communication as currently used falls short of this ideal. Reviews of the literature also concur with the general opinion. Thus the literature can offer specific advice to clinicians in practice who wish to improve their written communication. Some research has contrasted the personal opinions of GPs and specialists on what constitutes ideal written communication with analysis of existing written communications [9, 19].

22.4   How Do Patients, Doctors and the General Public View Each Other's Communication?

22.4.1 Mutual Perceptions of Dialogue Between Specialist Doctors and General Practitioners

There is some disagreement between GPs and hospital specialists about how ideal their respective letters are. Hospital specialists regard GPs' letters as insufficiently detailed and consider that their advice on management is often not heeded. GPs, for their part, feel that the hospital specialists fail to adequately deal with questions they are asked. A Dutch study took opinions from a cross-sectional sample of GPs and hospital specialists chosen at random from the Netherlands Medical Address Book [20]. There were 550 GPs and 533 hospital specialists involved. The survey results indicate that only 32.8% of hospital specialists felt GPs could be readily contacted by telephone to provide feedback, whereas GPs themselves put this figure at 85.3%. The hospital specialists were typically disappointed in the quality of referral documentation from primary care, with only 29.1% of specialists considering this paperwork of a good standard. Meanwhile, only 1 in 2 GPs were satisfied their questions were fully answered by specialists, whereas the specialists rated their own performance considerably better. Similarly, GPs felt they followed specialist advice more frequently than specialists thought. Less than 25% of GPs felt that written communication from the specialist arrived in a timely fashion, whereas specialists again rated this factor more highly. Both sides reported a wish for feedback from the other, but this seldom appeared to occur [20]. In terms of quality of written communication, 78.6% of secondary care letters were rated as excellent, whereas primary care referrals were rated as excellent in only 39.5% of cases [18]. It was found that the medication details in primary care referrals were deficient (either wrong items or incorrect doses) 42% of the time [21]. A Norwegian study used the Delphi method with two panels of experts consisting of a secondary care specialist, primary care physician and public health nurse. Letters sent to refer patients and discharge them from a single, general hospital facility were evaluated via a standard protocol in which ratings were recorded on a visual analogue scale [22]. The experts evaluated how well the presenting condition was described, the background medical history, physical examination, drug history, ability to carry out daily living activities, degree of social support, requirement for domiciliary care and whether care in hospital would be advantageous. The results indicated significant disagreement between primary and secondary care physicians and that referral letters were mostly inadequate, which raised the risk of medical mishaps. One in five discharge documents lacked essential medical details and not even 50% of discharge documents had adequate detail on daily living abilities, social support or the need to supply domiciliary care. Interestingly, 11% of secondary and 28% of primary care physicians considered their own documentation of inadequate quality, usually citing time pressure as the cause [9, 11].

22.5 Specific Documents Used to Communicate

22.5.1 Referral Letters to Secondary Care from Primary Care Physicians

In a study undertaken over two decades ago, Newton et al. asked both secondary and primary care physicians what should be included in a referral letter. In most cases there was considerable agreement [16]. This study also examined the expectations from a referral by primary care physicians. Tattersall et al. [23] discovered, by contrast, significant disparity between the views of primary and secondary care physicians about the expected informational content. This study also evaluated GPs' expectations from referrals.

22.5.1.1 Replies from Secondary Care, Including Discharge Documentation Following Admission to Hospital

Kripalani et al. looked at which items GPs felt were the most needed in discharge documentation to enable the patient to be followed up satisfactorily in primary care. The following lists the items primary care physicians expected, followed by the percentage of documents where this was missing in parentheses: principal diagnosis (13–17.5%); results of physical examination (10.5–45.5%); investigations and their outcome (38–65%); test results still awaited when the patient was discharged (65–88%); drug details at the point of discharge (21–25%) together with an explanation for any alterations; follow-up plan (14–30%) and information provided to the patient and carers (91–92%) [24]. A study predating Kripalani's showed that secondary care physicians rarely (less than 20% of letters) comment on the patient's social situation [25]. It has been noted that incorrect diagnoses may be written in discharge documentation, and the drug history recorded may not tally with the discharge medications supplied to the patient (in 39% of cases) [26]. Tattersall et al. undertook a comparison of letters intended for patients on discharge and those intended for the referring primary care physician. The letters to the referring primary care physician had gaps concerning further investigations needed, alternative therapeutic options, adverse effects and clinical prognosis [27].

22.6 Timely Communication

Several researchers have evaluated how timely the communication between physicians is, both in terms of how timely it appears subjectively and in quantitative terms. There is little doubt that communication occurs more effectively when there is no delay in transmission, from the point of view of all parties [9].

Alongside the inadequately informative nature of many physician letters, delays in transmission are commonly cited as an issue in healthcare communication. Primary care physicians cite delay in communication as a grave issue [28, 29]. Not even 1 in 4 GPs considered letters from secondary care to arrive on time, despite 61.8% of secondary care physicians believing they were usually timely in communicating [20]. Seven days after a patient had been discharged from hospital, only 53% of discharge documentation had arrived in primary care, and around 1 in 9 letters failed to arrive altogether. Accordingly, it was common for patients themselves to advise their primary care physician that they had been in hospital, since, in between 16 and 53% of cases, the discharge documentation was delayed [24]. There are a number of reasons why communication is so tardy, related to the processes involved, such as a delay in the secondary care physician composing the document (either by word processing or dictating it), slowness in typing dictated letters and delayed signing by the clinician [20]. The complexity of the process may account for the differences in how timeliness is perceived by primary and secondary care physicians. Secondary care physicians state that they reply to primary care colleagues in under a week, but primary care physicians state that such a reply only reaches their hands 36% of the time [11]. Furthermore, 1 month following an appointment in secondary care, a quarter of the primary care physicians were still awaiting a response from the specialist [11].

When communication occurs inefficiently in healthcare, a number of possibly harmful outcomes may occur, affecting all parts of the system. If communication fails, patients cannot be offered joined up (ideally seamless) healthcare, since each part then operates according to its own rhythm. The continuity necessary to provide quality healthcare applies especially to integrity of the information held. In chronic diseases, there needs to be a complete record of what has already occurred and how the disease and treatment are progressing [30]. Clearly, possessing information about previous history helps clinicians to choose more appropriate treatment plans, whilst the absence of such information may cause untoward events or actual harm to patients. Inefficient communicative practices can also result in delayed consultations, setting of appointments, recognition of disorders and slow management of conditions [9, 31, 32].

22.7   Recommended Ways to Optimise Communication in Writing

22.7.1 Letter Structure

Many authorities suggest that letters passing between primary and secondary care should follow a structured format. Secondary care letters might, for instance, have a section listing current problems, the suggested treatment and some fields for free text commentary. A structured format in documentation improves the understanding of the reader without lengthening reading time [33]. Discharge documentation following a template is generally better in quality and shorter than usual [34] whilst also preferred by primary care physicians. Despite this, secondary care physicians following a template are in the minority [35]. Primary care referrers may be able to nudge secondary care colleagues towards a more structured format by posing specific enquiries in the referral, prompting a reply following the format of the original referral [9, 36].

The greater utilisation of a structured communication format is helped by digitisation of clinical documentation [37]. An even greater advance may be accomplished if the system prompts a structured reply rather than offering free text entry [38]. Advances in health informatics systems mean that some applications can generate letters according to a predefined template [39]. Most primary care physicians demonstrate a preference for such automatically generated correspondence, as it is clearer and more guaranteed to provide the necessary information [9, 40].

22.7.2 Use of Peer Feedback to Improve Communication

A further technique which may improve the quality of healthcare communication is to solicit feedback on clinical communications. Primary care physicians may ask secondary care colleagues to feed back on the strengths and weaknesses of referral letters, allowing communication to become more targeted, following adjustment [41]. Naturally, this process can be enacted in reverse for secondary care letters. It has been shown that written communication becomes higher quality following peer-to-peer feedback [36, 42]. There are specific methods which can be employed to make the best use of feedback [9, 12].

22.7.3 Change Management Aspects

It is vitally important that written communication between primary and secondary care physicians be of high quality. As Durbin et al. have noted, change management in the healthcare system is very difficult. It may be more effective to aim for a broad change of culture or approach than to focus narrowly on a single outcome. It has been suggested in a review of audit practice in mental healthcare organisations that the most effective results are obtained through use of guidelines, training and structured documentation [31]. Automatically producing clinical documentation through the use of an application is very different from dictating letters to be transcribed by a secretary. The software produces the letters in a more timely fashion (assessed as letters prepared within 4 weeks of discharge) whilst simultaneously ensuring that vital information is unlikely to be left out [43–46]. Primary care physicians can also benefit from auto-generated referral documentation, which lowers the time spent on administration and may result in fewer delayed letters [9, 11].

22.8   Results Linked to Communication Quality

22.8.1 Accuracy of Diagnoses

The majority of the data needed to reach an accurate diagnosis are usually gathered during the patient history [47]. Despite the centrality of a good history in management, research has repeatedly shown that patients are granted too little time or attention to provide a high quality history. This situation frequently results from the consultation being interrupted. An inadequate history threatens the accuracy of the diagnosis, and, since the whole management of the patient depends on such data, wrong decisions become more likely.

Interrupted consultations give the patient the impression that their explanation carries little weight and makes them decide to withhold additional facts, which may influence subsequent management. In other words, allowing a consultation to be interrupted means a loss of valuable data and is detrimental to the doctor–patient therapeutic alliance [3].

22.8.2 Compliance with Treatment

Patients who are compliant with treatment act to follow the advice and recommendations provided by a doctor or other healthcare professional [48]. Non-compliance with treatment is widely recognised to present a significant barrier to success in managing many cases. The Health Care Quality Survey undertaken by the Commonwealth Fund established that a quarter of patients in the USA were not compliant with the clinician's recommended course of action [49]. The following were the reasons cited for non-compliance [3]:

- In 39% of cases, the patient had a different idea from the doctor about the best treatment approach.
- Concern about economic impact was cited by 27%.
- The instructions given were too complex for 25% of patients to follow.
- The treatment plan conflicted with personal beliefs in 20% of cases.
- Some 7% of patients reported not knowing what the treatment plan actually was.

22.8.3 Factors Making Patients Feel Satisfied

The central factors leading patients to feel satisfied include the following [50]:

- *Meeting the patient's expectations* by giving the space necessary to say what occurred.
- *Communicating Well:* Patients felt more satisfied when healthcare professionals engaged with their care gave importance to the issues, provided informative replies to questions, attempted to empathise and offered a genuine set of treatment alternatives.
- *Allow Patients to Feel in Control*: Patients who are given the opportunity to talk about their own views, worries and hopes have higher levels of satisfaction.
- *Involvement in Decisions*: Patients felt more satisfied if attention was paid to their social roles and mental health alongside physical health concerns.
- *Length of Consultation*: There was a correlation between longer appointments and patients feeling more satisfied.

- *Other Members of the Healthcare Team:* Patient satisfaction is most influenced by how they see their doctor. However, other team members also play a role in how satisfied patients feel.
- *Referrals to Other Professionals:* Patients expressed relief when a healthcare team took on responsibility for referring a patient, rather than leaving it up to the patient.
- *Continuous care* increased patient satisfaction. Patients do not enjoy being passed from doctor to doctor.
- *Dignified Treatment:* As could be anticipated, doctors who treat patients in a dignified way and include them in decision-making as a partner have more satisfied patients.

22.8.4 Patient Safety

It has been estimated that 1 in 3 adverse events are the result of either human error or a faulty system [51]. Studies undertaken for the decade from 1995 to 2005 concluded that two-thirds of medical errors arose from a failure of communication in medical teams. Therefore, if healthcare professionals do not practise effective communication, this will often have a detrimental effect on how patients are cared for. The likelihood of a clinical error goes up if clinical teams are placed under increased stress, have increased volumes of work or when communication lacks clarity or effectiveness [51].

22.8.5 Why Is It Important for Teams to Feel Satisfied?

It is important for healthcare teams to experience satisfaction for a number of reasons. The way members of teams in healthcare communicate with each other has a significant impact on relationships at work, the degree to which their job provides satisfaction and deeply affects the safety of patients [51]. Teams which communicate effectively regarding workload and responsibilities have been shown in studies to have lower rates of turnover for nurses [52] and higher rates of their members feeling satisfied at work. This effect is the result of effective communication fostering an environment where colleagues are mutually supportive [53]. Furthermore, as Larson and Yao showed [54] doctors who are good at establishing rapport with patients and are caring and warm in their interactions are much more likely to feel satisfied by their working life.

References

1. Clark PA. Medical practices' sensitivity to patients' needs: opportunities and practices for improvement. J Ambul Care Manage. 2003;26(2):110–23.

2. Wanzer MB, Booth-Butterfield M, Gruber K. Perceptions of health care providers' communication: relationships between patient-centered communication and satisfaction. Health Care Commun. 2004;16(3):363–84.
3. Impact of communication in healthcare. https://healthcarecomm.org/about-us/impact-of-communication-in-healthcare/. Accessed 11 Mar 2022.
4. Duffy FD, Gordon GH, Whelan G, Cole-Kelly K, Frankel R. Assessing competence in communication and interpersonal skills: the Kalamazoo II report. Acad Med. 2004;79:495–507.
5. Heisler M, Bouknight RR, Hayward RA, Smith DM, Kerr EA. The relative importance of physician communication, participatory decision-making, and patient understanding in diabetes self-management. J Gen Intern Med. 2002;17:243–52.
6. Renzi C, Abeni D, Picardi A, Agostini E, Melchi CF, Pasquini P, Prudu P, Braga M. Factors associated with patient satisfaction with care among dermatological outpatients. Br J Dermatol. 2001;145:617–23.
7. Safran DG, Taira D, Rogers WH, Kosinski M, Ware JE, Tarlov AR. Linking primary care performance to outcomes of care. J Fam Pract. 1998;47(3):213–20.
8. Sullivan LM, Stein MD, Savetsky JB, Samet JH. The doctor-patient relationship and HIV-infected patients' satisfaction with primary care physicians. J Gen Intern Med. 2000;15:462–9.
9. Vermeir P, Vandijck D, Degroote S, Peleman R, Verhaeghe R, Mortier E, Hallaert G, Van Daele S, Buylaert W, Vogelaers D. Communication in healthcare: a narrative review of the literature and practical recommendations. Int J Clin Pract. 2015;69(11):1257–67.
10. Solet DJ, Norvell JM, Rutan GH, Frankel RM. Lost in translation: challenges and opportunities in physician-to-physician communication during patient handoffs. Acad Med. 2005;80:1094–9.
11. Gandhi TK, Sittig DF, Franklin M, et al. Communication breakdown in the outpatient referral process. J Gen Intern Med. 2000;15:626–31.
12. Francois J. Tool to assess the quality of consultation and referral request letters in family medicine. Can Fam Phys. 2011;57:574–5.
13. Thorsen O, Hartveit M, Baerheim A. General practitioners' reflections on referring: an asymmetric or non-dialogical process? Scand J Prim Health Care. 2012;30:241–6.
14. Understanding oral and written communication. GeekInterview.com. 2011. http://www.learn.geekinterview.com/career/communication-skills/understanding-oral-written-communication.html. Accessed 7 Mar 2014.
15. Campbell B, Vanslembroek K, Whitehead E, et al. Views of doctors on clinical correspondence: questionnaire survey and audit of content of letters. BMJ. 2004;328:1060–1.
16. Pixy Ferris S. Writing electronically: the effects of computers on traditional writing. J Electronic Publ. 2002;8 https://doi.org/10.3998/3336451.0008.104.
17. Jacobs LG, Pringle MA. Referral letters and replies from orthopaedic departments: opportunities missed. BMJ. 1990;301:470–3.
18. Westerman RF, Hull FM, Bezemer PD, Gort G. A study of communication between general practitioners and specialists. Br J Gen Pract. 1990;40:445–9.
19. Newton J, Eccles M, Hutchinson A. Communication between general practitioners and consultants: what should their letters contain? BMJ. 1992;304:821–4.
20. Berendsen AJ, Kuiken A, Benneker WH, et al. How do general practitioners and specialists value their mutual communication? A survey. BMC Health Serv Res. 2009;9:143.
21. Carney SL. Medication accuracy and general practitioner referral letters. Intern Med J. 2006;36:132–4.
22. Garasen H, Johnsen R. The quality of communication about older patients between hospital physicians and general practitioners: a panel study assessment. BMC Health Serv Res. 2007;7:133.
23. Tattersall MH, Butow PN, Brown JE, Thompson JF. Improving doctors' letters. Med J Aust. 2002;177:516–20.
24. Kripalani S, LeFevre F, Phillips CO, et al. Deficits in communication and information transfer between hospital-based and primary care physicians: implications for patient safety and continuity of care. JAMA. 2007;297:831–41.

25. Bado W, Williams CJ. Usefulness of letters from hospitals to general practitioners. Br Med J. 1984;288:1813–4.
26. Adhiyaman V, Oke A, White AD, Shah IU. Diagnoses in discharge communications: how far are they reliable? Int J Clin Pract. 2000;54:457–8.
27. Tattersall MH, Griffin A, Dunn SM, et al. Writing to referring doctors after a new patient consultation. What is wanted and what was contained in letters from one medical oncologist? Aust NZ J Med. 1995;25:479–82.
28. Farquhar MC, Barclay SI, Earl H, et al. Barriers to effective communication across the primary/secondary interface: examples from the ovarian cancer patient journey (a qualitative study). Eur J Cancer Care. 2005;14:359–66.
29. McConnell D, Butow PN, Tattersall MH. Improving the letters we write: an exploration of doctor-doctor communication in cancer care. Br J Cancer. 1999;80:427–37.
30. Haggerty JL, Reid RJ, Freeman GK, et al. Continuity of care: a multidisciplinary review. BMJ. 2003;327:1219–21.
31. Durbin J, Barnsley J, Finlayson B, et al. Quality of communication between primary health care and mental health care: an examination of referral and discharge letters. J Behav Health Serv Res. 2012;39:445–61.
32. Epstein RM. Communication between primary care physicians and consultants. Arch Fam Med. 1995;4:403–9.
33. Melville C, Hands S, Jones P. Randomised trial of the effects of structuring clinic correspondence. Arch Dis Child. 2002;86:374–5.
34. Rao P, Andrei A, Fried A, et al. Assessing quality and efficiency of discharge summaries. Am J Med Qual. 2005;20:337–43.
35. Rawal J, Barnett P, Lloyd BW. Use of structured letters to improve communication between hospital doctors and general practitioners. BMJ. 1993;307:1044.
36. Grol R, Rooijackers-Lemmers N, van Kaathoven L, et al. Communication at the interface: do better referral letters produce better consultant replies? Br J Gen Pract. 2003;53:217–9.
37. Prince SB, Herrin DM. The role of information technology in healthcare communications, efficiency, and patient safety: application and results. J Nurs Admin. 2007;37:184–7.
38. Kern LM, Dhopeshwarkar R, Barron Y, et al. Measuring the effects of health information technology on quality of care: a novel set of proposed metrics for electronic quality reporting. Jt Comm J Qual Patient Saf. 2009;35:359–69.
39. Wasson J, Pearce L, Alun-Jones T. Improving correspondence to general practitioners regarding patients attending the ENT emergency clinic: a regional general practitioner survey and audit. J Laryngol Otol. 2007;121:1189–93.
40. Ray S, Archbold RA, Preston S, et al. Computer-generated correspondence for patients attending an open-access chest pain clinic. J R Coll Physicians Lond. 1998;32:420–1.
41. Jiwa M, Walters S, Mathers N. Referral letters to colorectal surgeons: the impact of peer-mediated feedback. Br J Gen Pract. 2004;54:123–6.
42. Keely E, Myers K, Dojeiji S, Campbell C. Peer assessment of outpatient consultation letters–feasibility and satisfaction. BMC Med Educ. 2007;7:13.
43. Sandler DA, Mitchell JR. Interim discharge summaries: how are they best delivered to general practitioners? Br Med J. 1987;295:1523–5.
44. Lissauer T, Paterson CM, Simons A, Beard RW. Evaluation of computer generated neonatal discharge summaries. Arch Dis Child. 1991;66:433–6.
45. Smith RP, Holzman GB. The application of a computer data base system to the generation of hospital discharge summaries. Obstet Gynecol. 1989;73:803–7.
46. van Walraven C, Laupacis A, Seth R, Wells G. Dictated versus database-generated discharge summaries: a randomized clinical trial. Can Med Assoc J. 1999;160:319–26.
47. Peterson MC, Holbrook J, Von Hales D, Smith NL, Staker LV. Contributions of the history, physical examination and laboratory investigation in making medical diagnoses. West J Med. 1992;156:163–5.
48. World Health Organization. Adherence to long-term therapies: evidence for action. Geneva: WHO Library Cataloguing. World Health Organization; 2003.

49. Davis K, Schoenbaum SC, Collins KS, Tenney K, Hughes DL, Audet AM. Room for improvement: patients report on the quality of their health care. New York: Commonwealth Fund; 2002.
50. Thiedke CC. What do we really know about patient satisfaction? Fam Pract Manag. 2007;14(1):33–6.
51. Team strategies and tools to enhance performance and patient safety (TeamSTEPPS). Department of Defense and Agency for Healthcare Research and Quality. http://www.ahrq.gov/qual/teamstepps/.
52. Lein C, Wills CE. Using patient-centered interviewing skills to manage complex patient encounters in primary care. Am Acad Nur Practition. 2007;19:215–20.
53. DiMeglio K, Lucas S, Padula C. Group cohesion and nurse satisfaction: examination of a team-building approach. J Nurs Adm. 2005;35(3):110–20.
54. Larson EB, Yao X. Clinical empathy as emotional labor in the patient-physician relationship. J Am Med Assoc. 2005;293(9):100–1106.

Online vs Face-to-Face Presentations: Advantages and Disadvantages

23

23.1 Introduction

A dictionary definition of the word "meeting" offers "an assembly of people for a particular purpose", indicating that, at the time of definition, the lexicographer did not consider the possibility of virtual meeting but instead saw the face-to-face aspect as intrinsic to the definition. However, as communication systems have evolved and developed, virtual meetings have sprung up in response to a perceived need. The main driving force behind such online meetings was the physical distance separating the participants and the impossibility of holding an actual face-to-face gathering, as often occurs in multi-national companies. The COVID-19 pandemic also meant many face-to-face meetings were replaced by online sessions to reduce the risk of disease transmission. Indeed, so essential was it to reduce the risk of viral transmission that even people working in adjoining rooms or offices opted for virtual meetings in place of physical gatherings. Although there was considerable initial reluctance by many to taking part in virtual meetings, necessity meant that many people were obliged to learn how to join such meetings. After they got used to the differences between the two types of meetings, they accepted them as a feasible alternative to conventional face-to-face gatherings.

So, what exactly is an "online" or "virtual" meeting? The terms are essentially used interchangeably. As with any meeting, a virtual meeting is undertaken to achieve some objective, but expands the possibilities by reducing the usual barriers to meeting for individuals in different locations, namely the physical separation and the time and cost of travelling to a common venue. An online meeting can be conducted at any time and location. For this reason, online meetings have enjoyed considerable attention in the commercial, academic and other fields. This chapter, therefore, aims to examine the differences between virtual and actual meetings, pointing out the advantages and disadvantages of carrying out meetings online [1].

Online communication and presentations utilise the VoIP protocol to transfer audio, and thus participants typically can choose between loudspeakers or

C. C. Cingi et al., *Improving Online Presentations*,
https://doi.org/10.1007/978-3-031-28328-4_23

239

headphones for listening to the meeting. When a presentation is given online, it is easy for the session audio and/or video to be recorded for future reference by anyone interested in the presentation [1].

23.2 Virtual Presentations

Online presentations may be audio-only or a combination of video plus audio (i.e. videoconferencing). Audio-only teleconferencing is efficient and inexpensive if there is a need to supply a select group of people with the same information at the same time. However, if the audience becomes too large or the audio quality is not high, this method becomes an ineffective way of communicating. Normally, people rely on visual clues to decide when to speak and when to listen, as well as to understand what is being said [2].

Videoconferencing is therefore rapidly becoming the default standard for online meetings, thanks to its ability to facilitate effective and efficient communication. Various applications are available for use in videoconferencing, such as Zoom, Polycom and Google Chat. The people involved see video of each other and can freely pass on their information and opinions, with the presenter well-placed to understand who is asking a question and where to direct his or her remarks. Not only do videoconferences work out cheaper both in direct economic costs and in terms of time involved, the attendance level is typically higher than in face-to-face events, and those participating benefit from a more equal balance between time spent at work and time available for home and leisure pursuits. Anyone who misses the session can watch the recording and presentations can be recycled for use in training and education [2].

Although it is straightforward to arrange a virtual meeting or presentation, for an effective outcome appropriate equipment must be selected and planning undertaken [2].

23.2.1 The Advantages of Virtual Presentations

23.2.1.1   The Ability to Communicate

All types of co-operative endeavour call for virtual conferencing capabilities. By using the specialised teleconferencing applications available, participants can easily communicate with each other, whether they are in the same building or in locations thousands of kilometres apart.

Teleconferencing applications can connect people in ways that allow a powerful connection to be formed and for results to be achieved.

Virtual meetings can go ahead even when events that cause disruption (freak weather conditions, war, pandemics, etc.) occur. They provide continuity in communication.

For these reasons, virtual meetings are currently considered one of the most effective ways for people to communicate with each other [1].

23.2.1.2 Ease of Access

Meetings which require attendance at a single venue may be difficult for individuals spread out over various locations internationally.

When individuals are physically present at a meeting, the costs rise. Thus, virtual meetings have a lower cost barrier.

In a virtual conference, people do not need to travel to participate. The conference is literally within arms reach [1].

23.2.1.3 Economies of Time

Another important aspect in which virtual meetings offer benefit is that they use up less of the participants' time. From a commercial viewpoint, time must be paid for. Thus, any measure which can spare this valuable resource is an advantage and helps the business to achieve its objectives. The time saved by doing the meeting online translates into more capital for investment.

Not only do virtual meetings save *some* time, they actually save *a vast amount* of time. Attendees no longer need to travel, to stay in another city and to plan their trip and spend time purchasing tickets.

Virtual meetings are not restricted by the availability of a venue and allowing time for attendees to arrive. The sole requirement is usually a reliable method for getting online, i.e. connecting to the internet [1].

23.2.1.4 How Cost-Effective Are Virtual Meetings?

It is prudent for any organisation needing to hold meetings to maximise the return on investment. One side of achieving this is minimising costs. Virtual meetings offer substantial savings on travel costs and the price of attendees staying in hotels, etc.

Moreover, the meeting itself entails direct costs when conducted face-to-face. The venue must be paid for and refreshments are usually expected by the attendees. These direct costs do not apply if the meeting is held online [1].

23.2.1.5 Improved Rate of Attendance

Individuals who join an online meeting do not spend their time travelling, hence the time commitment required is much less. Furthermore, it is more convenient and much less disruptive for participants to mute their microphones and/or switch their cameras off to answer an urgent enquiry than to step out of a face-to-face meeting.

These features of virtual meetings give the participants extra flexibility, which then means they are more motivated to participate in scheduled meetings, rather than sending their apologies on the grounds of being too busy [1].

23.2.1.6 Information Sharing

It is common practice to provide participants at face-to-face meetings with printed copies of the agenda and any related documentation. In virtual meetings, this seldom occurs, since electronic copies can be easily consulted when sitting at a laptop.

Because the meeting materials are distributed in electronic format, there are savings both in printing costs and the time required to wait for the items to be printed [1]. No extra copies requiring confidential disposal are required.

23.2.2 Disadvantages of Virtual Presentations

23.2.2.1   Reduced Personal Contact

The optimal form for humans to communicate with each other is face-to-face. The reason for the superiority of this communicative mode is that body language and facial expressions provide additional meaning to messages. The expression on someone's face deepens the significance of the message, whilst communication where facial expression cannot be observed is more prone to result in misunderstandings. Virtual meetings prevent this deeper form of communication and mean that important aspects of communication may be missed.

For example, healthcare professionals often engage in case discussions where there is some unclarity about the true diagnosis or potential disagreement about the optimal approach to manage that case. In such a detailed and important discussion, missing body language clues due to not communicating face-to-face may lead to important omissions.

23.2.2.2   Unstable Connection

It would be naïve to utilise technology in a way that ignored the possibility of cyber-crime, including fraud. Likewise, never assume that the internet connection will remain stable throughout an entire meeting. Indeed, it is not unusual for a connection to get dropped at least once during a meeting.

Unfortunately, dropped connections or loss of signal during an online meeting may make the event less effective, whatever the nature of the presentation. If this sort of problem occurs regularly, it may indicate the need for a router or other equipment to be updated [1].

23.2.2.3   Reduction in Human Contact

Not every face-to-face event can be successfully replicated by an online meeting. Some degree of socialising is needed to keep a close relationship working. Unfortunately, videoconferencing tends to remove the element of socialisation from events and removes much of the warmth from relationships.

Videoconferences tend to focus exclusively on business matters, removing the opportunity for wider-ranging conversations amongst the participants [1].

23.2.2.4   The Danger of Security Breaches

Virtual meetings involve a high risk of security being compromised. If cybercriminals target a meeting, they may be able to steal commercial secrets or other sensitive information, which they can then sell on or otherwise misuse. Because of these risks, participants in online meetings should follow strict security protocols regarding electronic transfer of information [1].

23.2.2.5   Inadequate Planning

Virtual meetings are much more straightforward to organise than many face-to-face events. There is no need to reserve a physical venue, arrange payments and print copies of the meeting materials, for example.

Nonetheless, for a meeting to achieve its objectives, the event still needs to be carefully planned in advance. Organisers of online meetings should be careful not to fall into the trap of believing a virtual meeting requires only minimal planning. The type of planning for virtual events differs from that needed for face-to-face events, but careful consideration is still needed [1].

23.3 Face-to-Face Presentations

Face-to-face meetings offer networking opportunities and the chance for personal engagement. Coffee break discussions, socialising events and conference meals help teams to establish themselves. When attendees are at a face-to-face event, they tend to be less easily distracted from the business of the meeting than may occur with an online event. Both the presenters and the audience members can read many body language clues which reveal how engaged they are with the topic and what their feeling may be. These clues can be lost with videoconferencing. Teams tend to trust each other more when they have actually met in person [2].

Conversely, meeting face-to-face may be simply impossible for some attendees, since it involves too great a financial cost, time commitment and opportunity cost. Finding a slot when each potential attendee is not already committed to something else may prove highly challenging. Not only is scheduling difficult for face-to-face meetings, there is also the need to factor in the cost and effort of travelling to and from an event, plus the possibility that unfavourable weather conditions, strikes, etc. will make travel unfeasible [2].

23.3.1 Aspects in Which Face-to-Face Meetings Have the Advantage

- Attendees can easily co-operate to resolve any issues.
- There is a high level of inclusion.
- The whole group can be brought onboard a new project.
- Some attendees find working as a group less stressful or demanding than needing to work individually. Unfortunately this may lead some less-motivated employees to sit back and let others do the work.

23.3.2 Disadvantages of Face-to-Face Meetings

- These meetings entail a high opportunity cost.
- Some people attend because they are invited, not because they have anything to contribute.
- Some meetings are dominated by the personalities of the individuals involved, rather than the agenda.

- Meetings where minutes are not recorded are frequently unproductive as nobody accepts responsibility to take action [3].

23.4   Comparison of Virtual and Face-to-Face Meetings

- Face-to-face meetings generally involve the need to provide pens, notepads, flip charts, refreshments, etc., whereas virtual meeting software provides all the facilities required automatically.
- Face-to-face meetings can be easily disrupted by other employees, whereas in a virtual meeting an attendee can answer an urgent call without disrupting the flow of the meeting.
- Some attendees at face-to-face meetings may get into the habit of using a meeting as a time to avoid other work or may fail to concentrate on the topic, as meetings may seem to blend into each other when they are very frequent.
- A possible third option alongside face-to-face meetings at the usual venue and virtual meetings is to hold the event at a different location. These kinds of meetings are often preferred when there is a need for face-to-face interactions but without the distractions of the everyday business. They may be called "offsite" meetings. Whereas a face-to-face meeting in the usual place of work ("onsite meeting") may seem mundane, an offsite meeting may break the routine and energise the attendees to come up with innovative ideas and rethink their assumptions [4].

23.5   Blended Meetings

One way to combine the benefits of virtual and face-to-face meetings or presentations is to create a "blended" meeting. This can be achieved in several different formats. There may be an initial virtual event after which a face-to-face gathering is arranged, or a speaker who would normally be unable to attend, through other time commitments or travel difficulties, may attend via videolink. This format lets the meeting benefit from the natural synergy that face-to-face meetings tend to generate whilst also benefiting from the flexibility and ease of organisation of virtual meetings [2].

Of course, as with all types of meetings, blended meetings are not a panacea. If an audience is very large, perhaps 200 individuals, communication is likely to be almost entirely unidirectional. A video-linked key speaker may easily communicate in this way. However, interaction with such a large audience may be very difficult, as the remote speaker may struggle to know who is asking a question or expressing an opinion. Nonetheless, for smaller audiences, say up to 30 individuals, there can be effective blending of the remote speaker with the natural dynamics of the face-to-face audience [2].

References

1. Advantages and disadvantages of online meetings. My own conference. 2020. https://myown-conference.com/blog/en/advantages-disadvantages-online-meetings/. Accessed 11 Mar 2022.
2. On-site vs. virtual meetings. 2019.https://hutchinsoncenter.umaine.edu/2019/06/28/on-site-vs-virtual-meetings/. Accessed 11 Mar 2022.
3. Skloot G. Advantages and disadvantages of meetings. https://getweeklyupdate.com/blog/advantages-and-disadvantages-of-meetings/. Accessed 11 Mar 2022.
4. Onsite v. offsite meetings. https://www.blueoceanfacilities.com/latest-blog/onsite-v-offsite-meetings/. Accessed 11 Mar 2022.